PRINCIPLES

OF

INTENSIVE

PSYCHOTHER

# PRINCIPLES

OF

# INTENSIVE

# PSYCHOTHERAPY

*Frieda Fromm-Reichmann, M.D.*

THE UNIVERSITY OF CHICAGO PRESS

CHICAGO AND LONDON

THE UNIVERSITY OF CHICAGO COMMITTEE
ON PUBLICATIONS IN BIOLOGY AND MEDICINE

LOWELL T. COGGESHALL · LESTER R. DRAGSTEDT
FRANKLIN C. McLEAN · C. PHILLIP MILLER
THOMAS PARK · WILLIAM H. TALIAFERRO

RC
480
F76

THE UNIVERSITY OF CHICAGO PRESS, CHICAGO 60637
The University of Chicago Press, Ltd., London

ISBN: 0–226–26598–6 (clothbound); 0–226–26599–4
(paperbound)
Library of Congress Catalog Card Number: 50–9782

80 79                    18 17 16 15

*To My Teachers*


SIGMUND FREUD

KURT GOLDSTEIN

GEORG GRODDECK

HARRY STACK SULLIVAN

# PREFACE

THIS book on principles of intensive psychotherapy represents an elaboration on a lecture course on the same topic which I presented to students of the Washington School of Psychiatry, the Washington-Baltimore Psychoanalytic Institute in Washington, and the William Alanson White Institute of Psychiatry in New York. The audiences were composed of psychoanalysts and psychiatrists in psychoanalytic training and other professional people engaged in psychiatric or psychological research and in practical professional work, which presupposes an interest and requires skill and knowledge in handling human relations.

It is upon the request of many of these students and following an invitation extended by the University of Chicago Press that these lectures have been prepared for publication. In its outline of the philosophy of the interpersonal principles involved, the book addresses itself, first, to psychoanalytically interested psychiatrists and to young psychoanalysts and, second, to serious students of living, such as were the members of the groups that attended the lectures for the purpose of increasing their skill in conducting interviews, in remedial work, and in interpersonal guidance.

It must be stated, though, that merely reading the book does not constitute a preparation for the practical application of the psychoanalytic principles outlined. Qualification for using them for therapeutic purposes must be obtained by special training in postgraduate psychiatric and psychoanalytic schools. Throughout the book, reference will be made to the nature of these indispensable training requirements.

In addition to the four great teachers to whom this book is dedicated, I wish to express my gratitude, above all, to my colleagues of the medical staff of the Chestnut Lodge Sanitarium and, furthermore, to the faculty members of the three schools, for stimulation received in discussions about all or many of the topics with which this book is concerned.

I am also indebted to my students, who taught me a great deal

[ vii ]

by their questions and suggestions in the classroom, in seminars, and in individual discussions of their patients, and to my own patients, who furnished the body of experience from which I drew while preparing the lectures and the book. (Where examples from patients' treatment histories have been offered, disguises have been used to veil their identity.)

Finally, I wish to express my special gratitude and appreciation to my friend and editorial secretary, Virginia K. Gunst, C.W.S.P., for her ever present readiness and indefatigable help in editing this book, in collecting the literature, and in preparing the Index and Reference List.

FRIEDA FROMM-REICHMANN

ROCKVILLE, MARYLAND
CHESTNUT LODGE

# INTRODUCTION

THIS book presents formulations of principles of intensive psychotherapy with psychoneurotics and psychotics. These psychotherapeutic principles are offered on the basis of a general dynamic and psychiatric orientation; more specifically, they are suggested to the reader on the basis of my training in and my experience with the application of Sigmund Freud's concepts of psychoanalytic psychotherapy with neurotics, the development of these teachings during the last fifty years, and especially of H. S. Sullivan's operational interpersonal conceptions. These doctrines form the background for my scientific orientation concerning the nature of and the procedure in intensive psychotherapy.

In view of the multitude of existing schools of psychotherapeutic thinking and so that the reader may roughly know what expectations to harbor about the content matter of this book, I will briefly define the guiding concepts of this discussion of intensive psychotherapy. The therapeutic procedure presented is intended to effect mitigation of a person's emotional difficulties in living and to bring about recovery from his mental symptoms. The psychotherapeutic process is designed to bring about understanding for and insight into the historical and dynamic factors which, unknown to the patient, are among the causes of the mental disturbance for which he seeks psychiatric help.

The technique used in this process is described in detail throughout the book. Very briefly outlined here, it comprises: the clarification of a patient's difficulties with his fellow-men through observation and investigation of the vicissitudes of the mutual interrelationship between doctor and patient; the encouragement of recall of forgotten memories; the investigation and scrutiny of the anxiety connected with such recall, including the patient's resistance against this recall and his security operations with the psychiatrist who tries to effect it. It is in the light of these memories and of the patient's and doctor's interpersonal experiences with each other that the patient's communications are interpreted with regard to their unconscious genetic and dynamic implications.

[ ix ]

The goal of intensive psychotherapy therefore, as I see it and as it is viewed by those to whom this book is dedicated, is understood to be: alleviation of patients' emotional difficulties in living and elimination of the symptomatology, this goal to be reached by gaining insight into and understanding of the unconscious roots of patients' problems, the genetics and dynamics, on the part of both patient and psychiatrist, whereby such understanding and insight may frequently promote changes in the dynamic structure of the patient's personality.*

This therapeutic goal of intensive psychotherapy is in contradistinction to the aim of other important psychotherapeutic methods and techniques, such as brief psychotherapy, suggestive psychotherapy, hypnotherapy, etc. Their goal is to cure symptoms and effect social recoveries. They operate without promoting personality changes and without producing insight into the genetics and dynamics of a patient's problems, or they center upon only a limited focal amount of insight.

Throughout the book I have used many examples. They are offered in an effort to illustrate the functioning of the psychotherapeutic process and various aspects of the psychotherapeutic interchange between patient and psychiatrist. It is my intention to exemplify that it is *not only the wording per se* (i.e., the interpretive give-and-take) which relieves the patient but also the discharge of affect plus insight gained by the patient. The nonverbal interplay experienced between patient and doctor which accompanies verbalized interchange also plays an integral part in all intensive psychotherapy. Therefore, verbatim statements of patient and doctor are quoted not only because of the logical contents which they convey but equally because of their interpersonal affective connotations.

A description of some of these indispensable affective concomitants to the psychotherapeutic process is included in the general discussion of the doctor-patient relationship in the part

* From this formulation of "intensive psychotherapy" my psychiatric philosophy becomes evident: that there is no valid *intensive* psychotherapy other than that which is psychoanalytic or psychoanalytically oriented. For this reason the reader will find that the term "psychiatrist" is used throughout this book in reference to the doctor who is engaged in psychoanalytic or dynamically oriented intensive psychotherapy.

on "The Psychiatrist" (pp. 3–42). Others are discussed in the sections on "Transference and Parataxic Distortions," "Security Operations, Resistance," and "Acting Out." Further manifestations of the ever present affective interpersonal elements of the psychotherapeutic process unfortunately defy accurate scientific description at the present state of our knowledge of and skill in accounting for these intangibles of the interpersonal interchange. The aim of special research projects now under way in the Washington School of Psychiatry and the Chestnut Lodge Sanitarium is to seek insight into and to discover methods to remedy these limitations.

It may surprise some readers to find that as many of these examples have been selected from my experience and that of my associates with seriously disturbed patients (psychotics) as from our work with neurotics. This seemingly diverse selection is initially motivated by the conviction which I share with H. S. Sullivan (149) that the progress and development of psychoanalytic psychotherapy with all types of patients has been greatly enhanced by the more recent experiences in psychoanalytic psychotherapy with psychotics. I will account for this belief, first, in this Introduction and again in the chapter on "Interpretation and Its Application" (pp. 80–84).

Further justification for my not discriminating between the use of experiences gained in the treatment of the more serious mental disorders of the psychotic and those of the milder forms of problems in living of the neurotic stems from another conviction. It is my belief that the problems and emotional difficulties of mental patients, neurotics or psychotics, are, in principle, rather similar to one another and also to the emotional difficulties in living from which we all suffer at times. Should these difficulties become so great that a person is unable to resolve them without help, thereby feeling the need for assistance, he may become a mental patient in need of psychotherapy.

I have put this statement at the beginning of this book because of my firm belief that the first prerequisite for successful psychotherapy is the respect that the psychiatrist must extend to the mental patient. Such respect can be valid only if the psychiatrist realizes that his patient's difficulties in living are not too different from his own. This statement is not just a humanitarian or charitable hypothesis but a scientific conviction. There are various well-known psychiatric facts which point in this direction.*

The first of these is the two-sidedness of motivation which the modes of expression of the so-called "healthy" have in common with many modes of expression of the mentally disturbed, as they present themselves in their symptoms. Many emotional reactions of both mentally disturbed and mentally stable people are an expression of a continuous or transitory disturbance of their emotional stability in terms of difficulties in their interpersonal relationships as well as an expression of their motivation toward alleviating or overcoming these difficulties. For instance, consider an obsessional person suffering from compulsive handwashing. He has to wash his hands from fifteen to thirty times daily, each time he touches certain things or persons from which he fears contamination. This compulsion is a mental symptom which seriously interferes with the maintenance of the person's interpersonal contacts. However, were he not to give in to the compulsion, his fear of contamination, which he fights with his compulsive handwashing, would interfere even more seriously with his contacts with other people.

Another example would be a withdrawn, aloof, seclusive schizophrenic. His aloofness constitutes a serious interpersonal difficulty. At the same time, it is motivated by a tendency to forego even more serious interpersonal difficulties. As one patient put it, it may be meant to forego "another rebuke," in the long row of thwarting rebuffs which the schizophrenic has experienced in his early childhood and which have conditioned him to expect repetition (67). Or it may serve the purpose of avoiding the outbursts of hostility against other people by which so many schizophrenics feel threatened within themselves.

Now, consider any average so-called "healthy" person who suffers from anxiety, that is, from a very unpleasant interference with his interpersonal contacts. Since he lives in a society and in a culture where the display of fear or anxiety are coexistent with an alleged or real decrease of prestige or self-respect, he may tend to

* Although I have elaborated upon them in a previous publication, I will repeat them here because of their bearing upon the attitude of respect between the psychiatrist and the mental patient.

convert his anxiety into anger, preferably against the person who is the cause of his anxiety. While this anger is an expression of a transitory interpersonal difficulty, it is, therefore, also the expression of a tendency toward alleviating this difficulty if and when it is masked as anxiety (54).

Again, consider a healthy person who is given to boasting and bragging to cover up his sense of inferiority. Pseudo-megalomanic outbursts certainly constitute a nuisance in our interpersonal world. However, the feelings of inferiority for whose overcompensation these outbursts are staged, constitute a much more serious interpersonal interference, that is, transitory difficulty in living. The realization and display of lack of self-respect will always be accompanied by a reduction of one's respect for others and therefore by the expectation of a decrease of the respect which one may expect from others. "One can respect others only to the extent that one respects oneself," as H. S. Sullivan put it (58, 104, 147).

So much for the two-sidedness of motivation which prevails equally in many emotional reactions of mentally disturbed and mentally healthy people. The other type of psychological expression which is evidenced by mentally healthy, as well as by mentally disturbed, people are the means of expression used by the mentally healthy while asleep, in their dreams, and by the mentally disturbed while awake, in their psychotic productions. Dreams and psychotic productions are actually analogous. To mention only a few of the operations common to them, both the dreamer and the psychotic express themselves in allusions, symbols, and pictures and by means of distortions and condensations. Both experience illusions and hallucinations. In both states, thinking does not follow the rules of logic, and the sense of time and space are not congruent with the chronological and topographical concepts of time and space which are valid with the healthy while awake (52, 89, 147). In brief, the psychotic operates along the lines of thinking and uses the means of expression with which the psychiatrist, who is familiar with the principles of psychoanalytic dream interpretation, is well acquainted (cf. "Dreams," pp. 161–73). Considered from the aspect of teleological thinking, one may even say that dreams follow the same pattern of two-sidedness in motivation as do other emotional experiences mentioned above. The dream constitutes, as it were, a transitory psychotic state through which we all pass once within a period of twenty-four hours. Some psychiatrists feel that it may be assumed that, in doing so, we safeguard against the danger of developing continuous psychotic states while awake. So much to corroborate the statement about the similarity in operation of the emotional difficulties of mental patients and those of healthy people.

What, then, is the nature of these difficulties? Emotional difficulties in living are difficulties in interpersonal relationships; and a person is not emotionally hampered, that is, he is mentally healthy to the extent to which he is able to be aware of, and therefore to handle, his interpersonal relationships (147). In stating this and, by implication, defining psychiatry and psychotherapy as the science and art of interpersonal relationships, I not only wish to say that a person is mentally healthy to the extent to which he is able to be aware of and to handle his overt relationships with other people. But I also wish to refer to a much more far-reaching fact. We can understand human personality only in terms of interpersonal relationships. There is no way to know about human personality other than by means of what one person conveys to another, that is, in terms of his relationship with him. Moreover, the private mental and emotional experiences, his *covert inner* thought and reverie processes are *also* in terms of interpersonal experiences.

From this interpersonal concept of psychiatry it ensues that intensive psychotherapy comprises the investigation and understanding of a person's overt and covert mental operations as interpersonal processes. Neither of these processes can be scrutinized or understood other than in terms of a person's interpersonal exchange with another person, be it in reality, as in overt relationships, or in fantasy, as in one's thought—and reverie—processes. When the experience is a psychotherapeutic one, it is the interpersonal exchange between the patient and the psychiatrist as a participant observer which carries the possibility of therapeutically valid interpersonal investigation and formulation.

We assume that it is true that emotional problems in general and the symptomatology of a mental patient in particular are due to difficulties in interpersonal relationships, for which there is reduced awareness. Subsequently, then, the principal problem of the psychotherapeutic interview is to facilitate the accession to awareness of information about interpersonal problems and difficulties which will help to clarify for the patient the troublesome aspects of his life and ultimately to resolve his symptomatology (147). This information must be sought with the patient and given by him as communication to another person, the psychiatrist. Hence it follows that the psychotherapeutic process is of a strictly interpersonal nature as to procedure and as to contents.

As we set out to investigate and clarify the principles of intensive psychotherapy, we must study, therefore, not only the psychotherapeutic process as such, or the patient's personality in terms of his interpersonal processes, but also the personality of the participant observer, the psychiatrist, in terms of his interpersonal relationships.

# TABLE OF CONTENTS

# TABLE OF CONTENTS

# PART I

## THE PSYCHIATRIST: PERSONAL AND PROFESSIONAL REQUIREMENTS

# CHAPTER I

## Insight into the Emotional Aspects of the Doctor-Patient Relationship

THE average psychiatrist who has acquired some knowledge of the principles of intensive psychotherapy has, by and large, studied only the psychotherapeutic process and the problems concerning the patient's personality. Unless he has undergone psychoanalytic training, not much attention has been given to the investigation of his own personality. Unless the psychiatrist is widely aware of his own interpersonal processes so that he can handle them for the benefit of the patient in their interpersonal therapeutic dealings with each other, no successful psychotherapy can eventuate.

It is to the immortal credit of Sigmund Freud that he was the first to understand and describe the psychotherapeutic process in terms of an interpersonal experience between patient and psychiatrist and that he was the first to call attention to and study the personality of the psychiatrist, as well as that of the patient and their mutual interpersonal relationship. Only those psychiatrists who have done psychotherapy both before and after being acquainted with Freud's concepts will be able to realize the full extent of the significance of his discovery of the laws governing the interpersonal exchange between doctor and patient. I personally remember only too well the time when I dealt psychotherapeutically with mental patients, before I was acquainted with Freud's teachings. I realized, with distress, that something went on in the patients' relations with me, and in my relations with them, which interfered with the psychotherapeutic process. Yet I could not put my finger on it, define it, or investigate it. What a relief it was to become acquainted with the tools furnished by Freud for investigation into and awareness of the doctor-patient relationship! Prior to these discoveries psychiatrists had been in the dark both to the detriment of their patients and to the disadvantage of their professional self-respect (38, 39, 40, 41, 46).

The debt of gratitude to Freud for his discovery of the need to study the doctor-patient relationship, in regard to the patient's as well as the doctor's part in it, still holds true regardless of the fact that Freud and his disciples subsequently nullified part of its far-reaching implications. As we know, Freud taught that all our relationships with other people, including the relationship of the mental patient with his doctor, are patterned by our early relationships with the significant people of our environment in infancy and childhood. Our later interpersonal difficulties have to be understood in terms of these early interpersonal tie-ups. The vicissitudes of the patient's experiences with the doctor, in particular, have to be investigated and understood for psychotherapeutic purposes. Since they are transferred, that is, carried over from unresolved difficulties in interpersonal relationships with the significant people of the patient's early life, they are "transference" experiences.

In the same way, the countertransference experiences of the doctor, as they, in their turn, come up and interfere with the psychotherapeutic process, must be investigated, understood, and, if possible, eliminated in terms of their being transferred from the doctor's early interpersonal experiences with the significant people of *his* infancy and childhood.

It is true that the patterns of our later interpersonal relationships are formed in our early lives, repeated in our later lives, and can be understood through the medium of their repetition with people in general and through the mutual aspects of the doctor-patient relationship in particular. There is, however, danger in carrying this insight too far. At the present developmental phase of dynamic psychoanalytic psychiatry, we still believe that it is not only helpful but indispensable for psychotherapeutic success to study the patient's and the psychiatrist's mutual relationships in terms of their repetitional characteristics. But we keenly feel that this should not be done to the point of neglecting to scrutinize the reality of the actual experience between therapist and patient in its own right. This viewpoint is also inherent in Freud's original teachings. But his transference doctrine gave an opening to obviate the fact of the actual experiences between therapist and patient then and there. In practice, this at times has carried with it the danger of inducing therapists to neglect the significance of the vicissitudes of the actual doctor-patient relationship as opposed to its transference aspects.

To illustrate: After a long period of painful procrastination, a patient in all seriousness and sincerity finally succeeded in conveying to the therapist what he considered to be his actual central difficulty. Conditioned to listening to the patient's stream of irrelevant talk, which he had unsuccessfully tried to break through thus far, the psychiatrist was not alert to the importance of the information finally offered. The patient, feeling hurt, became desperate and angry, questioned the usefulness of the psychotherapeutic process, and proceeded to evince open hostility. It is true that the patient reacted in this way because of his being especially sensitive to signs of just such lack of alertness because of similar warping and thwarting experiences with a significant adult in his early life. The patient's awareness of these experiences could be awakened or increased by studying them as he transferred them to the psychiatrist. But was it not of equally great, or even greater, importance for him, and more so for the doctor, to realize and admit that the patient was justified in his desperate anger against the therapist himself? After all, the therapist had failed the patient in his professional obligations by his lack of alertness when the patient most needed his discerning attention.

It may also be true that the psychiatrist's special sensitivity to the patient's meaningless chatter, hence his failure in being alert to the changed contents of the patient's communication, could be due to a pertinent experience in his own childhood. Suppose the doctor as a child had had to listen to the endless inconsequential talk of an elderly grandmother, to the point of becoming unable in his early years to pay attention to any significant communication of hers or of any other person's, which may have been interpolated into grandmother's chatter. But the knowledge of this countertransference character of the therapist's blunder does not eliminate the necessity of realizing his professional failure as such.

Recently the significant vicissitudes of the psychiatrist's relationship to his patients has been brought increasingly into the focus of therapeutic attention. This holds true for its transferred and for its factual aspects (112). Every psychiatrist now knows that there must be a fluctuating interplay between doctor and patient. This inevitably follows from the interpersonal character of the psychotherapeutic process. The psychiatrist who is trained in the observation and inner realization of his reaction to patients' manifestations can frequently utilize these reactions as a helpful instrument in understanding otherwise hidden implications in patients' communications. Thus the therapist's share in the reciprocal transference reactions of doctor and patient in the wider sense of the term may furnish an important guide in conducting the psychotherapeutic process. I will elaborate further on this important topic in this and other chapters of the book.

To return to patients' transference reactions, there is another point of departure from Freud's original teachings about transference in the concepts of psychoanalytic psychotherapy as they are outlined here. This variance stems from the fact that our thinking does not coincide with Freud's doctrine of the ubiquity of the Oedipus complex, the positive (sexual) attachment to the parent of the opposite sex, with concomitant rivalrous hatred for the parent of the same sex. Consequently, we do not understand as a foregone conclusion that the difficulties of therapists in their relationships with patients and vice versa stem from, or are only a repetition of, their unresolved Oedipus constellations (109).

H. S. Sullivan has introduced the term "parataxis" instead of "transference" and "countertransference." Parataxic interpersonal experiences are distortions in people's present interpersonal relationships. They are conditioned by carry-overs of a person's previous interpersonal experiences prevalently from infancy and childhood but not always or necessarily from entanglements with his parents (147).

So much for this preliminary discussion of the concepts of transference and countertransference and parataxis in their relevance for the understanding of the interpersonal processes of the psychiatrist. They will be discussed further throughout the book, especially in the sections on "Transference and Parataxic Distortions" (pp. 97–107) and "Security Operations, Resistance" (pp. 107–18).

At this point they are mentioned only to facilitate the realization that the interpersonal processes of the psychiatrist as a private and as a professional person must be investigated and recognized both in regard to the possibility of their being distorted as "countertransference," as "parataxic" experiences, and equally so in regard to the present interpersonal situation. This is one reason for requiring a personal psychoanalysis as part of the training for doing intensive psychotherapy.

# CHAPTER II

*The Psychiatrist's Part in the Doctor-Patient Relationship*

## 1. LISTENING AS A BASIC PSYCHOTHERAPEUTIC INSTRUMENTALITY

WHAT, then, are the basic requirements as to the personality and the professional abilities of a psychiatrist? If I were asked to answer this question in one sentence, I would reply, "The psychotherapist must be able to listen." This does not appear to be a startling statement, but it is intended to be just that. To be able to listen and to gather information from another person in this other person's own right, without reacting along the lines of one's own problems or experiences, of which one may be reminded, perhaps in a disturbing way, is an art of interpersonal exchange which few people are able to practice without special training. To be in command of this art is by no means tantamount to actually being a good psychiatrist, but it is the prerequisite of all intensive psychotherapy.

If it is true that the therapist must avoid reacting to patients' data in terms of his own life-experience, this means that he must have enough sources of satisfaction and security in his nonprofessional life to forego the temptation of using his patients for the pursuit of his personal satisfaction or security. If he has not been successful in securing the personal fulfilments in life which he wanted and needed, he should realize this. His attitude toward the sources of dissatisfaction and unhappiness in his life must then be clarified and integrated to the extent that they do not interfere with his emotional stability and with his ability to concentrate upon listening to the patient. This is a second reason for making a personal psychoanalysis a training requirement for a psychiatrist. Additional reasons will be discussed later.

The statement that the patient should not be a source of satisfaction and security to the therapist is, of course, not in reference to their actual, overt dealings with each other, since it is considered common knowledge that the professional relationship between psychiatrists and patients precludes any sort of nonprofessional mutual intimacy. What I am referring to is the danger that the discontented psychiatrist may use in fantasy the data collected from the patient as a substitutive source of satisfaction.

For example, a patient may tell a therapist who has just experienced an unhappy love relationship about problems of a similar nature. The psychiatrist should be sufficiently detached from his own problems so that he does not relate himself to the patient's experience and indulge in an orgy of self-referral. Or: a woman psychiatrist, who has passed the menopause and who regrets having only one child, hears about the third or fourth pregnancy of one of her patients. There should be no preoccupation with the denial of her own wishes intruding into her concentration upon the patient's report of her pregnancy. Again: a patient relates to the psychiatrist the progress in a happy courtship. Having in mind the lack of glamour in his own life, the psychiatrist may use the patient's review as one might use fiction or screen romance, namely, as a starting point for fantasies of his own. This fantasied projection of himself into the role of the patient or the patient's partner prevents the doctor from concentrating exclusively upon listening to the patient in his own right.

The same sort of experience may take place when a patient relates success or failure in prestige in any field. Whenever wishes or ambitions, fulfilments or failures, similar to those in the psychiatrist's career are touched upon, he must avoid the danger of using the patient's narrative as a starting point for dream satisfactions of his own, rather than using its narration as a source for collecting further helpful data about the patient. Although this ultimate goal has already been stated in the Hippocratic oath, the psychiatrist will only rarely be able, of course, to fulfil this ideal. Should he be unable to do so, he is expected to be aware of it, so that he can safeguard against the possibility of undesirable therapeutic consequences. This holds true for fantasies in the realm of both satisfaction and security.

In speaking about "satisfaction" and "security" as the two goals of fulfilment which man pursues, I follow H. S. Sullivan's definition (147). Satisfaction, he says, is the result of fulfilments in the realm of that which has to do with the bodily organization, the glandular processes, the need for sexual gratification and sleep, and the avoidance of hunger and physical loneliness. Security refers to the fulfilment of what has to do with the cultural equipment of a person, whereby the word "cultural" refers to everything which is man-made. Security, then, means fulfilment of a person's wishes for prestige, that is, the acceptance by and the respect of society as well as the achievement of self-respect. Security also means a person's being able to use successfully his powers, skills, and abilities for interpersonal goals within the range of his interests. *impact on others*

*Big*

## 2. THE PSYCHIATRIST'S NEED FOR EXTRA-PROFESSIONAL SOURCES OF SATISFACTION AND SECURITY

How, then, does the therapist's need for satisfaction and security have bearing upon his ability to listen, in addition to the previously discussed danger of allowing the material received from the patient to arouse his own fantasy?

Satisfaction of hunger has been mentioned as a necessary fulfilment; in our culture that means to have or to earn the money with which to buy food. The psychiatrist earns this money by means of his professional dealings with his patients. In that sense, practicing his profession is a legitimate source of satisfaction for him. What he has to safeguard against, however, is making psychotherapy with one patient the sole source of his satisfaction. In order to avoid having this happen, it is recommended that, in starting private practice, the young psychiatrist begin psychotherapy with two patients, or combine intensive psychotherapy with one patient with additional psychiatric activities of another type, such as part-time institutional work, teaching, consultations, etc. However unimportant this may seem to the inexperienced, psychotherapy with only one patient as the single source of income may easily be doomed to failure.

Sexual gratification has been quoted as another goal of satisfaction in man's life. The therapist has to safeguard strictly against using the patient, actually or in fantasy, for the pursuit of lust, so that sexual fantasies with regard to the patient or the partners whom the patient mentions, or identifications with the patient or his partners regarding their sexual experiences, do not interfere with the psychiatrist's ability to listen.

Obviously, man's need for sleep should not be sought by the therapist while attending to his professional obligations. But, unfortunately, I am giving away no secret when stating that there are therapists who fall asleep while they are supposed to listen, especially if they sit behind their patients and they do not see each other. There are even rationalizations on the part of psychiatrists for such unforgivable errors in procedure—such as "I only fall asleep if the patient produces irrelevant material and wake up as soon as the patient's productions become relevant." In marked contrast to such flimsy rationalization, I wish to emphasize strongly my viewpoint that the answer of the therapist to the patient's producing irrelevancies is not to take a nap but to listen sufficiently alertly so that he can interrupt and direct the patient toward the production of more relevant material. This statement implies a change of attitude with regard to the technique of "free associations" as used in classical psychoanalysis. I will elaborate on this topic later. If the psychiatrist indulges in napping during the psychotherapeutic interview, it interferes with his ability to listen and to conduct the interview adequately. It also has the implication of lowering the patient's self-respect as the doctor evidences how little interested he is in the patient and his communications. This may prove to be quite disastrous to the psychotherapeutic process, because the self-esteem of a psychiatric patient is very low to begin with. His lack of self-respect and his insecurity are, as a rule, wittingly or unwittingly, one of the reasons for his needing psychotherapy. One of the important principles of intensive psychotherapy to which I shall have to refer time and again is that the psychiatrist endeavor to improve patients' self-respect and that, by all means, he should avoid hurting it.

The classical psychoanalytic setup of the psychiatrist sitting behind the patient, who is lying on the couch, may imply the danger of encouraging any inclination on the part of the psychiatrist to drowse. At the time when the technique and methods of classical psychoanalytic therapy were developed, this position was considered desirable to induce a state of complete relaxation in the patient, which would make it possible for him to associate freely and to eliminate embarrassment while relating delicate and painful material. Moreover, the founder of classical psychoanalysis, Sigmund Freud, felt that he personally was not up to having patients look at him for eight hours daily, and he assumed that many of his colleagues might encounter the same difficulty (38).

Since then there has been a marked development in psychoanalytic insight and technique (93). Many psychoanalytic psychiatrists now feel that it is no longer necessary to listen to free associations over a long period of time in order to become acquainted with patients' psychopathology, and before administering any active psychotherapeutic intervention (5, 6). This is due to the increase in knowledge about the dynamics of mental processes which has been gained during the last fifty years. In addition, many topics, the communication of which was formerly fraught with extreme hesitancy and shyness, have gradually lost the connotation of embarrassment for most people in this culture during the last fifty years. Indeed, Freud's teachings are largely responsible for a more normal attitude toward the discussion of formerly prohibited sexual subject matter. Suggestions in technique, which he originally made to conform with the sensitivities of his contemporaries, are therefore now outdated by the very results of his teachings.

As to the hardship for the psychiatrist to be gazed at daily for eight hours, I believe that there were two reasons, both of which can be discounted today. One was that the therapist was liable to share the embarrassment of his patient while listening to difficult communications. The second was the original psychoanalytic concept, according to which the therapist was supposed to show no signs whatsoever of reacting to, or participating in, the patient's communications. The more colorless and the more inanimate the countenance of the psychiatrist appeared, the more nearly he approached the ideal of serving the patient as a recording machine on which he could record whatever was on his mind. This inanimate attitude also served as a safeguard against the psychiatrist's becoming personally involved with his patients and with the emotional experiences which they were reciting. The consistent control of facial expression, posture, and gestures which the psychiatrist had to exert under these conditions made it very hard indeed for him to be exposed to his patients' visual scrutiny all day long (63, 64).

Nowadays, many psychiatrists no longer think of the therapist as unresponsive to and only a mirror of the patient's utterances. We consider him a participant observer in the psychotherapeutic process. Also, we do not believe that it is necessary or desirable for the psychiatrist to bar responsive reactions of spontaneity from the psychotherapeutic scene, as long as his responsive facial expressions cannot be used by patients as a means of orientation inadvertently guiding their productions and behavior. Also they must, of course, be genuine responses to patients' communications and not colored by his private collateral experiences.

With these two concepts in mind, I consider it, by and large, much more desirable to have an arrangement which makes it possible for both the patient and the therapist to look at each other or not as the occasion may warrant. Prohibiting the use of visual contact as an aid in the therapeutic process is an unnecessary deterrent and makes for an unreal situation. This holds true especially for psychotic patients, whose lack of orientation in the outer world has to be counteracted by the visible and audible reality of another person. I will elaborate further on this topic while discussing the psychotherapeutic process (65).

As to the fourth goal of human satisfaction, the avoidance of physical loneliness, it goes without saying that the patient should not be used for its achievement. This does not mean advocating that the psychiatrist be an obsessional denizen of our culture, wherein touching another person or being touched by him is considered taboo unless there is an intimate relationship. The contrary is true. At times it may be indicated and wise to shake hands with a patient or, in the case of a very disturbed person, to touch him reassuringly or not to refuse his gesture of seeking affection and closeness. However, it is always recommended that one be thrifty with the expression of any physical contact.

A psychiatrist who is lonely must see that his own need for physical contact does not interfere with his coming to the correct conclusions about patients' needs. He must safeguard against a lack of alertness in listening due to this interference of his own unresolved needs.

Security operations should interfere just as little with the psychiatrist's ability to listen as should his personal needs for satisfaction. The psychiatrist who needs the individual patient to build up his prestige and to prove to himself that he is able to use his powers and his skills successfully will be in danger of trying to impress his patient instead of being impressed by the patient's needs and difficulties. This could hold true especially for the young psychiatrist, who might try to counteract his own insecurity in two ways which would interfere with his ability to listen. First, he might feel called upon to hide his insecurity by displaying professional pompousness. Such an endeavor is highly undesirable; in fact, it may doom the psychotherapeutic procedure to failure. As stated before, every mental patient suffers from an impairment in self-assurance, that is, he is insecure and anxious. This being so, he will be most sensitive to the attempts of another person to hide his insecurity. If this other person is his psychiatrist, the therapist's own ill-disguised insecurity will add to the patient's anxiety. The patient will not feel free to confide in the psychiatrist and to believe in his ability to listen; therefore, psychotherapeutic collaboration will be defeated.*

The young psychiatrist who may feel called upon to try to impress patients might keep in mind, furthermore, how unnecessary this is because the patients who come to see him want help. They expect him to be competent to offer this help on the basis of his training and/or because of his having been recommended by another successfully treated patient or by an older psychiatrist. Patients tend toward health, and they are lonely. Their wish for help, their tendency toward health, and their loneliness are much more important to them than the chronological or professional age of the person to whom they turn for aid.

The second way in which the psychiatrist may try to bolster his insecurity, namely, by cultivating the patient's dependence and admiration, is therefore equally unnecessary. This may interfere with the psychiatrist's ability to listen even more than the direct display of pompousness. The cultivation of such attitudes pushes

* Incidentally, psychiatrists who got their training in Central Europe and who are now doing psychotherapy in this country should keep in mind that their Anglo-Saxon patients will resent any display of pompousness even more than their European patients did.

his patients into a state of dependence, instead of working toward growth, independence, and an ability to use their own judgment. To put it differently, the psychiatrist duplicates the demands for unqualified love and acceptance of authority which the parents or other significant adults of the patient's childhood may have imposed on him to his detriment. In Freud's terminology, he artificially cultivates the patients' positive transference. As he does so, he can be reasonably certain that contrary results will be obtained in the long run. The patients will resent the psychiatrist's interference with their tendency toward and wish for growth and independence, since these are among the reasons for which they came to see the doctor, and they will hate their would-be helper for failing them. In other words, the psychiatrist's attempts at artificially cultivating his patient's positive transference will necessarily breed a negative attitude in the patient toward the psychiatrist.

Some unfortunate results of the need of the insecure psychiatrist to use the patient as a test tube for his skills and powers should be mentioned at this point. Such a psychiatrist may be so preoccupied with the idea that his patients have to get well for the sake of his reputation that he will listen to them and conduct treatment in such a way that he deafens himself against and disregards the patient's real needs and his striving for improvement. Or the insecure psychiatrist may feel that the patient must understand whatever the doctor feels called upon to point out, disregarding the question of whether or not the patient is ready to follow at the time. In the same vein, he may answer the patient's failure to understand with an intensified irritation, which, in turn, will certainly becloud the legitimate issues of the psychotherapeutic process. Moreover, the patient is liable to feel that he is being used as a means of confirming the psychiatrist's reputation rather than as an object of treatment in his own right. This attitude could well be conducive to the failure of treatment. In this connection, I recall the unhappy neurotic son of a powerful and influential father, whose life was dedicated solely to the increase of his father's prestige and reputation. He expected everyone with whom he came in contact to function only in order to impress his influential father or to be seeking prestige as his father did. Of course, the patient expected his psychiatrist to behave accordingly. "If I get well," he volunteered in his first interview, "it will be quite a feather in your cap." The psychiatrist was fortunately not preoccupied with his reputation, so that he heard the patient and the implications of his sarcastically polite remark. Much to the patient's surprise, he simply replied that his reputation was established to his satisfaction, independent of failure or success with any single patient. He added, as soon as the patient gave him an opening, that he was not interested in impressing the patient's father but solely in an attempt to be of use to the patient in his own right, if and when he cared for psychotherapeutic collaboration. Many years later, when the patient at last reached the goal of recovery, he dated the beginning of successful psychotherapy to this conversation.

Again, insecure psychiatrists may insist upon their patients doing and accomplishing things before they are ready for it. The patients may try to do so in an attempt to please and encourage their doctors, while they themselves become discouraged by the failure of their premature efforts. Most assuredly, the patient should *not* be put into the position of having to reassure the doctor. Fortunately, there are patients who are able to see and verbalize this danger. The psychiatrist who is not too preoccupied in his quest for gaining security at the expense of his patients may be able to hear their warning. This happened, for example, in the case of a catatonic patient whom the psychiatrist tried to push prematurely into resuming social contacts. The patient stated that she was on the road to recovery, even though social contacts were still repulsive to her. "Sometime in the near future," she remarked, "when I am convinced that no one is pushing me for ulterior motives, I will branch out under my own steam." Eventually, the psychiatrist heard the warning, even though it was not in line with the conventional treatment standards of the hospital and therefore derogatory to his prestige there. Had he continued pushing the patient into social contacts against her warning, he might have delayed, if not jeopardized, her recovery.

This admonition against the psychiatrist's pushing a patient in a certain direction for his own benefit should not be mistaken for a general cautioning against the therapeutic validity of any pushing of patients, sometimes against their own wish and conviction. In some types of patients whose cases will be discussed later, such active procedure is indicated and useful.

The preoccupation of the insecure psychiatrist with the need to assert himself at the expense of his patient has another unfortunate outcome: namely, the fantasy that the patient may be "clay in the hand of the builder" and that he can mold him according to his own image. Such wishes may lead the psychiatrist into fantasies about nonexisting similarities between him and his patients. These fantasies will make him resistive to obtaining a real picture of these patients' personalities and of their specific emotional difficulties in living. The patients will be expected to accept or work out the same solutions for their personal problems as those which the therapist has decided upon for his life. They will not get the help they need in searching for their own answers. In other cases, the patients are expected to accept the psychiatrist's set of personal values instead of being encouraged to find their own sets of values and to learn to follow them independently.

From these illustrative situations we can deduce the case in point: that the psychiatrist must have a reasonably stable self-esteem to avoid psychotherapeutic blundering. This offers another reason making it necessary for the psychiatrist to undergo a personal psychoanalysis before he undertakes intensive psychotherapy with others.

The following experience illustrates the beneficial significance ensuing for the patient if he finds his therapist to be a self-respecting person. A patient who had had to interrupt her treatment, because of moving to another city, returned after some time and asked the psychiatrist for an interview. The patient told him how disappointed she was with the results of her own treatment and with some failures of the psychiatrist which she had seen in other patients of his. She then expressed her doubts about his abilities at large and her resentment about his previous failure to warn her against overestimating him. The therapist discussed the patient's grievances and expressed regret about her remaining symptomatology. After that he said quietly and in a matter-of-fact way that he still considered himself a reasonably good psychiatrist. The patient was heard to utter a sigh of relief and responded by answering, "That is all I wanted to know." What she meant was that nothing mattered very much as long as she could rely upon the stability of her former therapist's self-respect.

There is one more reason why the psychiatrist's self-respect is of paramount significance for the therapeutic procedure. If it is true that one's ability to respect others is dependent upon the development of one's own self-respect, then it follows that only a self-respecting psychiatrist is capable of respecting his patients and of meeting them on the basis of mutual human equality. The self-respecting psychiatrist will keep in mind that he is in a superior category as compared with his patients only by virtue of his special training and experience, and not necessarily in any other way. His patients may or may not have greater personal assets than he has. To repeat what was said in the Introduction: the fact that a person needs psychiatric help in handling his emotional difficulties in living by no means constitutes any basic inferiority. Only the psychiatrist who realizes this is able to listen to his patients in such a way that there may be psychotherapeutic success.

The psychiatrist's respect for his patients will also help him to safeguard against the previously mentioned mistake of assuming an attitude of personal "irrational authority" instead of listening and conducting therapy in the spirit of collaborative guidance (56). This irrational authoritarian behavior will be harmful not only because it interferes per se with the patient's tendency toward growth and maturation but also, and more important, because it constitutes a traumatic repetition of the authoritarian aspects of the cultural pattern of behavior in general and of the parental pattern in particular, to which most mental patients have been harmfully subjected in their past (146).

This is not intended to rule out the psychiatrist's taking a firm and definite stand as an expert who establishes his "rational authority" in his psychotherapeutic suggestions. But it does rule out his taking advantage of the unhappy, intimidated, and overdependent patient's inclination to put him, as a person, on an authoritarian pedestal. For many psychiatrists the temptation to do so may be present as a means of getting even with annoying authoritarian domination to which they themselves have been subjected by their parents, teachers, or superiors and anonymously by society at large.

If the psychiatrist is self-respecting and has respect for his patients, his ability to listen will also not be impaired by fantasies of omniscience or perfectionism. He will realize that he is not called upon to be a magician who is expected to perform psychotherapeutic miracles. He will be able to admit mistakes, limitations, and shortcomings as they occur.

Insecure and self-righteous psychiatrists cannot endure their failure to understand patients' communications without developing feelings of anxiety or resentment. These psychiatrists cannot understand that the mental patient, who is supposed to be out of his mind, may say meaningful things which the psychiatrist, who is supposedly in his right mind, cannot understand.

This statement may seem redundant to those psychiatrists who work with ambulatory neurotics only. The psychiatrist who works with disturbed psychotics, however, will be faced time and again with his inability to follow the contents of the communications of his patients. This holds true despite the fact that psychiatrists learned from Freud to revise the teachings of classical psychiatry, which taught that most psychotic utterances made sense neither to the patient nor to the psychiatrist. It is not necessary, however, to understand all the patient's utterances. The disturbed patient, as a rule, does not mind if the therapist fails to understand the contents of his communications as long as the therapist is frank about it and does not make false pretenses. The therapist has to approach all of them, including the nonintelligible psychotic productions, the way he approaches the dreams of the healthy and of the neurotic. He expects to understand some of them and to be at a loss as to the meaning of others, yet he realizes that most of them are meaningful for the dreamer.

There was a time when we psychiatrists became overenthusiastic about the discovery of the potentially meaningful communications of our patients. This drove psychoanalytic psychotherapy into the false direction of concentrating on the contents of patients' communications and of overrating the psychotherapeutic usefulness of understanding them. This held true for the productions of the psychotic as well as for the inadvertent communications of the neurotic, his slips, and other phenomena, which Freud has described under the title of the *Psychopathology of Everyday Life* (49). That time has passed. We now consider the investigation of the origin, the timing, and the dynamics of neurotic and psychotic productions therapeutically more effective, without, of course, eliminating our interest in understanding the actual contents.

To illustrate: a hospitalized paranoid schizophrenic in her middle thirties, who had been overtly disturbed for thirteen years, started tending toward recovery after many months of intensive psychotherapy. One of her main symptoms until then had been the delusion of the appearance of "The Line." As yet the patient has not told the psychiatrist what "The Line" is; it may be she does not even know herself. However, she has succeeded, upon the inquiry of the therapist, in telling him each time what event preceded the appearance of "The Line," until they finally discovered what type of events in the patient's life created its appearance. "The Line" has now disappeared, and its elimination seems to have contributed greatly to the general improvement in the patient's condition.*

This example should remind the psychiatrist of two important facts. First, his interest in research should be secondary to his eagerness in discovering data strictly pertinent to his psychotherapeutic obligations. Second, he should not be pertinacious in searching for and in conveying understanding to the patient at the expense of observing what is going on in the patient. There is frequently no therapeutic advantage in doing so. As Freud said, "The psychoanalyst's job is to help the patient, not to demonstrate how clever the doctor is." Further elaboration on the significance of the origin and the dynamics of the patient's communications versus their contents will be incorporated in the discussion of the psychotherapeutic process.

The warning against psychiatrists' allowing fantasies of omniscience and perfectionism to interfere with their ability to listen and to admit such mistakes to themselves does not necessarily mean that the therapist should always feel obliged to admit his mistakes to his patients. The patient carries enough of his own worries without the therapist's increasing them, much less using his patient as father-confessor and thus burdening him further by an ill-advised concept of sincerity prompted by the psychiatrist's worry regarding his own mistakes. What really matters is that he be able

* For an elaborate study of this patient's history and treatment see Staveren, Ref. 143.

to admit his mistakes frankly to himself so that he can operate with insight.

On the other hand, there are times and situations when it is wise and therapeutically useful to comment on his errors to the patient in a matter-of-fact and nonmasochistic manner, as, for instance, in the following cases: A catatonic young man was very angry with his psychiatrist for unknown reasons. His rationalization was that the analyst was a foreigner with a marked accent. "Can't I have a physician who speaks decent English?" he exclaimed. He then became actively assaultive. About six weeks later, the patient was very pleased with some evidence of sensitive understanding on the therapist's part. "Aren't you from Cambridge?" he asked. The therapist did not grasp the implication that the patient desired to convey his wish to forgive the foreign accent by saying, as it were, "Your speech sounds as good as true Bostonian English." The psychiatrist, therefore, denied being from Boston and spoke of her native land and of her last European residence. The patient insisted that she must be from Cambridge, saying, "I am sure there was a girl from Cambridge, perhaps you have not been sufficiently introduced to her." Only after the psychiatrist had left the patient that day did the connection become clear to her between the interview of six weeks ago, when the patient scolded her because of her foreign accent, and today's interview, when he complimented her for her English. If a catatonic undergoes the risk of opening up sufficiently to ask forgiveness and to compliment the therapist, it has the connotation of a great gift. If the psychiatrist does not understand, thereby not accepting the gift, this may be experienced by the patient as a marked rebuke. Hence the psychiatrist felt that in this case it was indicated that she comment upon her failure to understand. At the next interview she told the patient that she had realized after they had seen each other what a fool she had been at their last session to give the patient the information about her background which he already knew, instead of having heard him say that he had ceased resenting his doctor's accent. The patient smiled and seemed to agree wholeheartedly with the psychiatrist's self-derision. The course of the interview confirmed the therapist's expectation regarding the beneficial result of admitting her failure.

Another example is taken from the treatment history of the catatonic girl about whom I have reported in my paper, "Remarks on the Philosophy of Mental Disorder" (70). This patient expressed her anxiety about her many months of hospitalization by telling the psychiatrist nearly every day that she should leave the hospital. She said that, if the doctors did not want her to leave, they owed her an exact statement about what, in their judgment, constituted her remaining illness. The psychiatrist acknowledged the legitimacy of this request and asked the patient to give her a day or two to think about a formulation which would be meaningful and useful to the patient. Then the statement was given, made sense to the patient, and was accepted. The next day, however, the patient again started expressing her wish to be dismissed. The psychiatrist was disappointed, became impatient, realized this, and felt that she should admit this failure, so she apologized. The patient expressed her appreciation of the recognition of failure on the part of the psychiatrist by stating that she felt it was up to her to apologize, not up to the doctor, as she had taxed the doctor's patience with her repetitional behavior. Patient and therapist were then able to agree upon the favorable aspects of a doctor-patient relationship in which both doctor and patient felt free to apologize to each other.

Sometimes it may be wise for the psychiatrist, should he anticipate difficulties which could arise from specific contrasts between his and the patient's personality makeup, to formulate this possibility to the patient, pointing out the danger of their interference with psychotherapeutic progress. The following experience exemplifies this. A very brilliant, clever, and shrewd psychopath, many of whose interpersonal relationships were in terms of power manipulations, was told after the first two interviews that the psychiatrist considered himself to be reasonably intelligent but much less clever and shrewd than the patient. The psychiatrist explained that it would be easy enough for the patient to put something over on him should he choose to use his superior shrewdness and cleverness for that purpose. It was then suggested to him that he try to make his choice between using the psychiatrist for what help he had to offer or as a target for his shrewd manipulations. In spite of this warning which the psychiatrist had offered for both the patient's and his own benefit, the patient succeeded more than once in deluding the psychiatrist during the course of the treatment. Since this was foreseen, it was easy to fall back upon the initial statement whenever it became necessary to disentangle any of the patient's shrewd, though unconstructive, power manipulations.

The psychiatrist's sense of security undergoes the greatest test of endurance when he is subjected to the mental patient's display of hostility. I am not in agreement with the teachings of classical analysis, according to which people are born to be hostile and aggressive, i.e., with Freud's teachings of the death instinct (43, 105). In this hostile world of ours, however, every person—certainly every mental patient—has sufficient reason for learning to develop reactions of hostility. Mental patients react with hostility to the hostile behavior and the shortcomings of the significant adults in their environment, including the failures of their therapist, and they transfer to him the anger and resentment engendered by their previous experiences. Furthermore, they interpret the therapist's behavior and communications along the lines of their unfavorable past experience with other people. Hence it follows that every mental patient will have to express a marked degree of hostility in the course of his interpersonal dealings with the therapist. This being so, psychotherapy can be successful only if the psychiatrist is secure enough himself so that he will be able to deal adequately with the hostile reactions of his patients.

There is another inevitable source of patients' hostile reactions against the therapist. This stems from the bipolarity in the dynamics of mental disorder. It was stated in the Introduction that mental symptoms are an expression of patients' anxiety. At the same time, they constitute a defense against anxiety, an attempt at warding it off. Patients' attitudes toward the psychotherapist are inevitably a reflection of this twofold meaning of their symptoms. The doctor who fights the symptomatology of patients is the object of these patients' friendly feelings, inasmuch as their attitudes are motivated by their inherent tendency toward regaining health. At the same time, mental patients will cling to their symptomatology because of its defensive quality. Therefore, the psychiatrist is also the target of their hostility, since his therapeutic endeavors are

[ 22 ]

aimed at depriving them of these defenses. Insight into the dynamic bipolarity of the symptomatology of mental patients should help the psychiatrist to endure these hostile outbursts, which are determined by the function and not by the personality of the therapist. Some psychiatrists seem to believe that they can exhibit their unadulterated willingness to listen constructively to patients' outbursts of hostility by inviting them, in so many words, to "express (their) hostility." This does not work, of course. First, one is not apt to follow any suggestion of a person toward whom one feels angry or resentful, much less the invitation to express one's resentment. Second, it is not likely to be followed because no one actually feels or thinks about his anger in terms of "hostility." The very use of this abstract term may make the patient feel that his anger, his rage, his fury, his resentment, etc., are minimized or not taken seriously when referred to as "hostility." Therefore, the psychiatrist who invites his patient to express (his) hostility, protects himself wittingly or unwittingly from becoming the actual target of this hostility.

Some therapists have learned to brace themselves in order to endure a patient's openly hostile onslaught, in a psychotherapeutically valid, that is, personally detached, way. These same psychiatrists, however, may not be able to live up to the professional standards in listening to their angry patients if this anger is expressed in the mitigated form of criticism of the doctor's personal or professional performances. Psychiatrists who do therapy with hospital or clinic patients may be tempted to argue away hostile invectives against their institutions. Since there may be a need to be loyal and defensive regarding the places with which they are connected, psychiatrists may blind themselves to the fact that, more often than not, patients may only seem to criticize or resent the hospital or the clinic. Actually, they may be using the institutions as targets for the expression of negative feelings which are directed against their therapist as part of this institution.

Another common way of being misled about patients' hostility or critical judgments stems from their complaints about other doctors who have treated them. The temptation to feel flattered by being considered better than the colleagues mentioned may induce the therapist to be inattentive to the fact that his colleagues are being used by the patient merely as a screen to express negative feelings or judgment about others when, instead, the patient is actually talking about his present psychiatrist.

The psychiatrist may feel his security all the more threatened by his patient's direct or veiled criticism if and when he feels that it is objectively justified. It is most desirable for a therapist to feel sufficiently secure, both as a person and in his work, that he may be able to listen and discern correctly justified and unjustified criticism. If he recognizes it as correct, he should be able to take it at its face value and to learn from it. If he considers it unjustified, he should be able to listen with his attention and his subsequent inquiries focused on the emotional reasons for the patient's needs to criticize.

Hypersensitivity to justified or unjustified appreciation or de-preciation of the psychiatrist's abilities, due to lack of self-respect, will particularly interfere with a therapist's constructive contacts with some groups of psychotics. Because of their marked anxiety, these people have developed a consistent watchfulness of their environment and great alertness regarding interpersonal experi-ences. Therefore, they are frequently capable of emotional eaves-dropping, as it were, on other persons, including their psychiatrist. From the gestures, attitudes, inadvertent words, and actions of the therapist, the psychotic may, at times, gain an empathic awareness of certain personality aspects of which the therapist himself may not be aware. Well-developed security is necessary for the therapist to be able to listen without resentment to his patients' comments on these more-often-than-not undesirable personality trends of which he may have been previously unaware.

### 3. INSIGHT INTO THE INTERACTION OF ANXIETY IN PSYCHIATRIST AND PATIENT

Where there is lack of security, there is anxiety; where there is anxiety, there is fear of the anxieties in others. The insecure psychiatrist is, therefore, liable to be afraid of his patients' anxiety. Hence he may not want to hear about their anxiety and their anxiety-provoking experiences. He may thwart the patients' tendency to submit these experiences to psychotherapeutic investigation by feeling called upon to give premature reassurance to patients because he needs reassurance himself. In doing so, he is liable to <u>obstruct his patients' verbalizations and the investigation of important emotional material.</u> Moreover, to the patient the psychiatrist's anxiety represents a measuring rod for his own anxiety-provoking qualities. If the therapist is very anxious, the patient may take that as a confirmation of his own fear of being threatening, that is, "bad." In other words, the therapist's anxiety decreases the patient's self-esteem (68).

A patient, for example, may tell his psychiatrist that he is afraid of his impulses to kill. The therapist, becoming fearful himself, may try to mitigate the patient's fear by some would-be reassuring, commonplace remark to the effect, for instance, that thought and action are not identical or that thinking of killing does not make one a murderer, etc. Hearing this, the patient will either realize that the doctor is *as* afraid if not *more* so than he is himself, and this realization will, in turn, increase the patient's fear; or he will assume that the doctor has no grasp of his actual fear of real destructive action. In either case the patient may feel barred from ever again verbalizing his terrible fright. If, however, the therapist shows the patient, by implication, that he appreciates the degree of the patient's anxiety, without becoming involved himself, he may be able to clear the road successfully for further therapeutic collaboration. He may, for example, make a constructive remark such as, "I wish you could tell me what hardship has come to you through other people in previous years that now makes you feel like murdering people" (69).

The statement that the psychiatrist should be able to endure a patient's hostile outbursts in word and action is by no means identical with the suggestion that he ought to grant every patient the freedom to express his hostile impulses at random. Many neurotics, especially hysterics, indulge in verbalized and play-acted hostile dramatizations, be it in overobedience to misinterpreted psychoanalytic writings or with the idea of testing the psychiatrist's endurance or of delaying constructive psychotherapeutic collaboration. In such cases the psychiatrist should interfere with the patient's display of hostility. Note, however, that he does so for the benefit of the patient and of the psychotherapeutic process, and not because of his own anxiety.

On the other hand, it is true that even psychiatrists with a reasonably well-developed sense of security may at times run into patients who evoke fear or anxiety in them. If the therapist is clearly aware of his own anxiety, he may be able to use it as a valid signpost in the direction of his understanding the meaning of the patient's anxiety-evoking communications which were otherwise hidden from him and from the patient. The therapist's anxiety may be aroused in connection with verbal reports about anxiety-producing material as well as in connection with actual acts of violence. The psychiatrist is liable to treat these patients along the line of his own anxieties, instead of facing the anxiety of the patient in a therapeutically valid manner.

In the case of threatening or real violence in action, the psychiatrist is justified and required to firmly express his unwillingness to be its target. He should also see to it that adequate precautionary measures are taken. This attitude is advocated not only for the sake of the doctor's own protection but just as much for the sake of the protection of the patient against actions the recall of which leads to self-derogation and self-depreciation.

In the case of the psychiatrist's anxiety being due to verbal productions or where there is failure to produce relief for himself by precautionary measures, the anxious psychiatrist should suggest to the patient that he change therapists and help him to do so, unless the doctor is able to discover unconscious reasons for his anxiety, which he is able to resolve psychoanalytically.

In a previous publication, I reported an impressive experience in point, to which I was submitted some years ago (69). A woman patient succeeded in making me afraid of her assaultiveness. It is true that she threatened repeatedly to hit me or to throw stones at me or get me jammed in the door as I entered or left the room; however, very little actually happened except for a few slaps in my face. I have worked with more dangerously assaultive male and female patients without being afraid. I knew, therefore, that there were irrational reasons for my fear of this patient. Since this anxiety interfered with psychotherapy and since I did not want to abandon the patient, I had a supervisory discussion regarding this negative countertransference of mine and became conscious of the reasons, upon which it subsided.

Here is a record of the interview which followed the supervisory discussion. I met the patient on the grounds of the hospital, and she greeted me, as usual, by shouting, "God damn your soul to hell," to which I responded, being now quite free of anxiety and fear, "For three months you have successfully tried to frighten me, yet neither you nor I have gotten anything out of it, so why not stop?" Patient: "All right, God damn your soul to . . . heaven!" Doctor: "That would not help either, because, if I died, I could not try to be of any use to you." By then, the patient had become aware of the fact that my fear, which, of course, had meant an offense to her, had gone. She bent to the ground, picked a flower, and handed it ceremoniously to me, saying, "O.K., let us go to your place and let's do our work there," which we did. The implication of the patient's request to take her to the office in my house was to test whether or not my fear of her assaultiveness had actually subsided. If I were still afraid, I would, of course, insist upon going to the hospital, where help against a patient's aggression would be more readily available than at my house. After this interview and my acceptance of her challenge, constructive psychotherapeutic collaboration between patient and doctor could be resumed.

In addition to the display of hostility in word and action, psychotic manifestations in general may arouse anxiety in some young psychiatrists. They may feel threatened by the fear of duplication within themselves of the psychotic symptomatology which they see portrayed before them.

If the psychiatrist has the good luck not to be afraid of psychotic patients and to be able to listen to their hostile outbursts without impairment of his sense of security, there will be two beneficial consequences. First, the very fact that the doctor does not become frightened will mitigate the patient's fear of his own aggression and therefore moderate his actual assaultiveness, which has been, in part, fear-born to begin with. Second, the psychiatrist's fearless reception of the patient's outbursts may lead to subsequent valid therapeutic developments, as in the following case of a very disturbed, assaultive, catatonic woman patient, who had been under treatment for one and one-half years without ever becoming assaultive toward the therapist. One day she came into the office and remained standing by the desk rather than taking a seat, as was her habit. Asked about the reason for this, she answered with considerable feeling, "You will admit that I have never done anything to you or to your things during all the time that I have come here to see you, no matter how upset I might have been. Today, I will knock all your things off the desk and then I will knock you down. You had better call your maid to protect you." Fortunately, the psychiatrist was not afraid, so that she was able to say, firmly and calmly, that she would not call anyone in for her protection. Had she asked for help against a patient who threatened assaultiveness but showed no real evidence of action, instead of concentrating upon the cause of this threat, she might easily have jeopardized the chances of further treatment. So the doctor decided to cope with the situation as follows: She realized, she said, that the patient could easily knock her down, should she choose to do so, since she was younger, stronger, taller, and more agile than the doctor. She hoped, however, that the patient would prefer to tell her about the reasons for her hostile mood. To this suggestion, the patient replied with great emphasis that this was not the time for her, an American-born woman, to discuss things with a (recently naturalized) German doctor. "Don't you know that there is a war on?" she continued. "The Americans and the Germans at the front do not talk things over, they fight." There followed another invitation to ask the maid in for the doctor's protection, then a suggestion on the doctor's part to the effect that the difference in the patient's and the doctor's nationality could not be the reason for the patient's fighting mood. The doctor reminded the patient of the fact that, in their previous contacts, she had never found the patient to be prejudiced in favor of Americans who had immigrated many generations ago rather than recently. She also mentioned that the patient had always known of the doctor's German origin and that previously this fact had not interfered with their psychotherapeutic interchange. The patient maintained her threatening attitude and posture for about three-quarters of an hour before giving in to the doctor's repeated, insistent requests to discuss the real reasons for her being upset.

Then, at last, the patient said with considerable feeling that one of the attendants on the ward had called her "a filthy, dirty homosexual." The psychiatrist immediately expressed her genuine concern and her intention to investigate and remedy the situation. The patient was now completely calm. She sat down, lighted a cigarette, and said, "It is no longer necessary to investigate the incident." She then looked at her watch, regretted the amount of time she had spent on her outburst of hostility, and suggested that at least the last few minutes of the interview should be used for serious psychotherapeutic work.

The basic cause for the patient's disturbance had not been merely the fact, which was later verified, that the attendant had called her a homosexual but that, from the implication of such abuse, the hospital and its staff considered homosexuality to be "filthy and dirty." To her this attitude was in direct contradiction to the therapist's initial statement during their first interview, that homosexuality was nothing of which to be ashamed or any reason for hospitalization, provided that it did not impair the patient's security of living among the average prejudiced inhabitants of this culture. Hence the attendant's abuse carried with it the connotation that the psychiatrist had been insincere when stating her own and the hospital's unprejudiced attitude regarding homosexuality. Therefore, the patient's emotional investment in the incident was immediately withdrawn as the psychiatrist divorced herself from any identification with the offender. The whole incident was subsequently utilized for a psychotherapeutically important investigation of the doctor-patient relationship with its implications regarding the patient's relationship with other people.

In order to illustrate some further reassuring features of the doctor's lack of fear of a patient's assaultiveness, I shall offer as an example an experience with a patient whom I have mentioned in a previous publication. I learned impressively from her about the dependence of patients' self-respect on the doctor's attitude. Because of her assaultiveness, she was seen in a pack for her interviews. One day I asked her, upon the superintendent's request, whether she would sign a check for us. (She was not committed; therefore, payments from her own funds for her stay in the hospital could only be made with her signature.) The patient declared that she would gladly sign the check if she were un-packed. As I went for the nurses to ask them to do so, some em-pathic notion for which I cannot give any account made me turn back toward the patient.* I saw an expression of utter despair and discouragement on her face, which made me decide to unpack her myself. After her recovery, she was capable of telling me that she considered my taking her out of the pack myself the starting point of her recovery. My doing so, in spite of her being much taller, heavier, and stronger than I, had the connotation for her that her doctor did not consider her to be too dangerous, that is, "too bad," to emerge from her mental disorder (66).

There is another therapeutically undesirable consequence of a psychiatrist's insecurity which can come from a handicap that plays a great role in the personality development and interpersonal attitude of many people; I mean the fear of being ridiculed. This fear is so universally characteristic of humanity because of the so-cial interrelatedness of its members that it is not infrequently used as a pedagogical deterrent by parents and teachers. As a matter of fact, there are some Indian tribes who use it as the only means of acculturating their children and of raising them to respect and accept the mores of the tribe (56).

The psychiatrist may be afraid of appearing ridiculous in the eyes of his colleagues or of the secretaries of his clinic. A patient may walk out on him or be markedly late for his interviews. The doctor may fear the ridicule of other patients or of the nurses on the ward, as a disturbed hospital patient soils his suit by throwing food at him, by spitting at him, by smearing feces on him, or if a patient locks the doctor in the room, etc. It would, of course, be desirable for the doctor to be able to overcome his fear of ridicule. Indeed, if he could, he would automatically take the wind out of

* "Empathy" is a term used by H. S. Sullivan, when referring to the emotional contagion or communion which exists between people outside the communication through sensory channels or through spoken words. I follow his thinking in the use of this term. He stated that empathy is first observed between infants and their mothers and that its greatest importance comes in late infancy and early childhood, from the age of six to twenty-seven months. In part it remains with us throughout life. My turning around to the patient is one instance of its functioning. Most readers will recognize it at work in certain interpersonal setups and at certain times and, quite use-fully so, in some instances of the psychiatrist's dealings with his patients (147).

the sails of those in whose eyes he fears to appear ridiculous. But it cannot be expected that he will always be able to conquer this fear. The quest for prestige in our culture is so great that it will interfere with some doctors' efforts to become desensitized to it. The trained psychiatrist, however, may be aware of his fear and try to work through it or, if unsuccessful, create a treatment setup which enables him to evade situations which threaten him with the sense of ridicule in the eyes of the environment.

# CHAPTER III

## The Psychiatrist's Attitude toward Cultural and Ethical Values in Its Relatedness to the Goals of Psychotherapy

THE need of an insecure psychiatrist to draw security from a virtuous adjustment to the conventionalities of his time and from a quest for approval from "the good and the great" may turn out to be another agent interfering with his ability to listen in a therapeutically valid fashion (66, 70). This type of dependence gives rise to the danger that the psychiatrist may consider the changeable man-made standards of the society in which he lives to be eternal values to which he and his patients must conform. Therefore, his ability to listen and to help will be limited, as his patients try to discover to what extent and in what way each of them needs to adjust to the cultural requirements of his time. He will be desensitized to the patient's personal needs because of preoccupation with his own dependency on the denizens of the society and culture of his era and its transitory values. As I have pointed out elsewhere, this may render him practically incapable of guiding certain types of patients: "The recovery of many schizophrenics and schizoid personalities, for example, depends upon the psychotherapist's freedom from convention and prejudice. These patients cannot and should not be asked to accept guidance toward a conventional adjustment to the customary requirements of our culture, much less to what the individual therapist personally considers these requirements to be. The psychiatrist should feel that his goal in treating schizoid personalities is reached if these people, without violating the law or hurting their neighbors, are able to find for themselves the sources of satisfaction and security in which they are interested. This presupposes, of course, that these patients have acquired, through inner freedom and independence from public opinion under the guidance of their psychiatrist, the ability to live their own lives irrespective of the approval of their neighbors" (68, 70).

In this connection, I am reminded of the girl about whom I have previously written. She recovered from a catatonic disturbance of eight years' duration, which time she had had to spend in mental hospitals. For many years now, this girl has been living in her own country home, stable, independent, and enjoying her household duties, her artistic accomplishments, and her friendly, casual, personal relationships and social activities. However, she did not fulfil the conventional criterion of a healthy adjustment for which this culture asks, namely, marriage. In spite of this, the therapist considered the goal of treatment reached.

On the other hand, there are, of course, many other types of patients, neurotics, for example, whose personalities are potentially in accord with the requirements and values of this culture. Their lack of adjustment is part of their symptomatology and should be subject to change through treatment. Many of them are eternal adolescents who refuse to grow up and who therefore try to maintain the defiant attitude of teen-agers toward that which represents to them the demands of the adults, against whom they rebel. These patients make it equally necessary for the therapist to be reasonably independent of social conventionality and evaluations in his own right, just as does the first group. Unless he is, there is danger of his becoming irritated by and defensive against the juvenile or adolescent rebellion of his adult neurotic patients, instead of recognizing it for what it is and treating it without undue emotional expenditure.

To summarize: security and inner independence of the authoritarian values attributed to the conventional requirements of our culture are indispensable for the therapist who wants to guide his patients successfully toward finding out about the degree of cultural adjustment which is adequate to their personal needs.

In early psychoanalytic literature, some authors claim that the psychiatrist should be free from any evaluational goals while dealing with his patients. To my mind, this holds true only for those personal evaluational systems of the psychiatrist which pertain to religion, philosophy, political viewpoints, and other questions of Weltanschauung, which he would not expect to be or to become the evaluational goals of his patients. It is not correct to say, however, that there is no inherent set of values connected with the goals of psychotherapy (57, 70, 73). Similar views are expressed by W. Riese in his manuscript: "Premiers principes d'une éthique médicale."

Treatment, of course, is aimed at the solution of the patient's difficulties in living and at the cure of his symptomatology. Ideally these therapeutic goals will be reached by the growth, maturation, and inner independence of the patient. Accomplishment will be further realized by his potential freedom from fear, anxiety, and the entanglements of greed, envy, and jealousy. This goal will also be actualized by the development of his capacity for self-realization, his ability to form durable relationships of intimacy with others, and to give and accept mature love. I define "mature love," in accordance with E. Fromm and H. S. Sullivan, as the state of interpersonal relatedness in which one is as concerned with the growth, maturation, welfare, and happiness of the beloved person as one is with one's own (58). This capacity for mature love presupposes the development of a healthy and stable self-respect (13, 58, 147, 162).*

By "self-realization" I mean a person's use of his talents, skills, and powers to his satisfaction within the realm of his own freely established realistic set of values. Furthermore, I mean the patient's ability to reach out for and to find fulfilment of his needs for satisfaction and security, as far as they can be attained without interfering with the law or the needs of his fellow-men. K. Goldstein's concept of "self-actualization" and E. Fromm's concept of the "productive character" cover what I have tried to establish here as the ideal goal of psychotherapy (57, 73; see also the section on "Termination of Treatment," pp. 188–94).

In the classical psychoanalytic literature, insufficient attention has been given so far to the concept of self-realization as a great source, if not the greatest source, of human fulfilment. Freud has referred to it in his teachings on secondary narcissism and ego ideal formations, but he has dealt more with the investigation of the origin than with the elaboration on the psychological significance of

* About Binswanger's philosophy of the *liebendes Beieinandersein* ("loving togetherness"), which is related to, but by no means identical with, these concepts, see Refs. 58 and 162. See also T. Benedek, Ref. 9a.

the phenomenon (47, 50). I will refrain from going into theory at this point and shall restrict myself to the emphasis on "self-realization" or "self-actualization" as a practical psychotherapeutic goal of paramount importance. Last but not least, the combined personality study and treatment which constitute psychotherapy should furnish the patient with the tools for the maintenance of his stability during periods of uncertainty, frustration, and unhappiness as they are bound to occur in everyone's life. The psychiatrist should not be afraid of being aware of these standards or to admit that these are the basic standards which guide him in his therapeutic dealings with his patients, no matter how eager he may be to establish his personal evaluational neutrality (68, 70, 147).*

Some psychiatrists set up the genital maturity of the patient as a criterion for his recovery, meaning his ability to be orgastically potent in heterosexual intercourse. They believe that the signs of recovery outlined here will accompany or result from genital matureness (129). I believe it to be the other way around. That is to say, a person who is reasonably free from anxiety, greed, envy, and jealousy and who is able to experience interpersonal intimacy will be capable of expressing this in terms of satisfactory sexual activities (169).

The suggestion that the psychiatrist be guided by these ethical goals of treatment is not intended to supersede my initial suggestion that he must safeguard against any interference with his professional attitude by his personal sets of ethical values in terms of matters of Weltanschauung. It is self-evident that this does not mean he should not verbalize evaluations to the patient. It should be emphasized, however, that ideally the psychiatrist keeps this type of personal evaluation sufficiently apart from his professional life to avoid their inadvertent emanation. The danger of the influence of such ever present and transpiring evaluational attitudes on the patient's development is increased by the specific state of the patient's emotional dependence on the psychiatrist for the duration

* Kubie (93) defines the goal of psychoanalysis in terms of the promotion of the following personality changes which are presuppositions for the goals of treatment as above defined: "Conscious dynamic adaptability and flexibility, . . . while creating and preserving an active need to eliminate the abuses in human life, coupled with clarity both about the reforming drive and about the abuses which demand reform."

of the treatment. This state of dependence per se makes the patient most sensitive to all his doctor's verbalized and nonverbalized communications. The dependence and alert sensitivity are increased by the laws governing the patient's relationship with the psychiatrist. They bring about the patient's tendency to transfer onto the psychiatrist the previous attitudes of dependence which he has felt toward those in authority in his past. Last but not least, they account for his tendency to interpret the doctor's actual utterances along the lines of past life-experiences with significant people. Rightly or wrongly, the patient will read, as it were, between the lines of what the therapist actually wishes to convey. The therapist must be prudent so as not to misuse the great sphere of influence granted him by his patients, much tempted though he may feel at times to use dependent attitudes of patients as a means of imbuing them with his own personal set of values. It would be quite easy to feel flattered by the patients' trust and dependence rather than to remain alert to the fact that their insecurity, hence overdependence, is part of the disturbance for which they seek treatment.

The emanation of the psychiatrist's general system of ethical values is not the only example of the possibility of inadvertent communication of his viewpoints and its influence on the course of the treatment. The emanation of the psychiatrist's evaluation of and judgment about the symptomatology of his patients may turn out to be of equally great importance. One of the most impressive examples illustrating this fact presents itself in the history of the psychiatric evaluation of the symptom of stool-smearing. In the old days, stool-smearing was considered to be a symptom of grave prognostic significance in any psychiatric patient. Since psychiatrists have learned to approach this symptom in the same spirit of investigating its psychopathology and its dynamics as they approach any other symptom or mode of expression, it has lost its threatening aspects. In other words, stool-smearing patients of previous periods in psychiatric development were sometimes destined to deteriorate and become incurable. This was not because of the inherent gravity of the symptom but because of the atmosphere of awe, disgust, and gruesomeness which it evoked in their moralistic, pedagogically minded psychiatrists and which they unwittingly conveyed to the patients (106, 142).

I have given one example to corroborate this viewpoint and ✓ quoted other authors who had similar experiences, in a previous publication (69). Here is one more example which stems from an ambulatory male schizophrenic. Hurt about a premature interpretation given to him in a previous interview by the psychiatrist, this patient opened the next interview with the following resentful statement. The psychiatrist had driven him to regress into infancy by his "wrong" interpretation. Upon coming home from the last interview, he started smearing his bowel movements all over himself and the bathroom walls and had continued to do so since then with great pleasure.

After having ascertained the legitimacy of the patient's resentment, the psychiatrist voiced his opinion that there must have been great relief and fun in defeating the old and severe taboo against stool-smearing. The patient expressed severe doubts of the psychiatrist's sincerity. Eventually he suggested that the therapist, if he meant what he said, join the patient in playing with his bowel movement, which he would deposit for that purpose on the office rug right then and there.

The doctor's reply to this was that he would do so if he considered it remedial—despite the fact that other people's bowel movements were more repulsive than one's own. However the doctor felt that he was engaged to help the patient to mature, not to join in his infantile play. Therefore, he felt that he should not follow the patient's suggestion. "This answer is of great therapeutic help," was the patient's immediate reply, to be followed at the next therapeutic hour by the report that he had stopped stool-smearing and that he found "intercourse to be better after all." This incident was followed by a marked improvement in the patient's general condition.

The inadvertent empathic conveyance to the patient of the psychiatrist's standards plays an important role in many more areas of the treatment situation. Many rules and regulations regarding the psychoanalytic setup have been established to facilitate the patient's and the psychiatrist's successful collaboration in intensive psychotherapy. These we will consider in detail as we come to the discussion of the psychotherapeutic process. It has been recommended that, by all means, one should avoid interruptions of psychotherapeutic interviews by actual interference or by accidental distractions, such as environmental noises. It has also been recommended that one make it a rule not to see one's patients outside the scheduled interviews, professionally or otherwise. These and other regulations are very helpful indeed in maintaining a therapeutically constructive doctor-patient relationship. The degree of good or evil consequences which result from violating these rules depends, however, mainly, if not solely, upon the degree of disturbance which such infraction creates in the minds of patient and therapist (41, 63, 64).

This becomes significantly understandable if one remembers how the same principle holds true in all our interpersonal relationships, beginning with the initial relationship between mother and infant. Much has been said, for example, about the time element in bowel training for children. We now know that it is not only the time element but the attitude of the mother who does the bowel training that is of paramount importance for the personality development of the child (72). By the same token, it is primarily the attitude of the psychiatrist who handles the rules and regulations governing the therapeutic interviews and only secondarily the maintenance or infraction of these regulations which make for the difference between psychotherapeutic success or failure.

# CHAPTER IV

## Considerations of the Psychiatrist in the Establishment of the Treatment Situation

BEFORE concluding the investigation of the psychiatrist's personal and professional requirements for correct handling of the doctor-patient relationship and the psychotherapeutic process, one more pertinent interpersonal problem of the psychiatrist must be mentioned: that is the question of the psychiatrist's like or dislike of a patient. Of course, it is his privilege to refuse acceptance of a patient for treatment if and when he feels he dislikes him as a person. Once he does accept the patient, however, these categories should be void of meaning in his professional dealings with patients. If a person comes to see the psychiatrist, this implies a need for changes in his personality; and if the psychiatrist accepts a person for treatment, this means that he recognizes that person's need for change and that he hopes to be instrumental in the patient's ultimate attainment of these necessary changes. This being so, the question of whether or not the patient in his present mental condition and with his present personality trends is to the psychiatrist's liking is beside the point.

The great significance which dynamic psychiatry contributes to the environmental factors and to the interpersonal traumata which help or interfere with the shaping of people's personalities is another fact which should happily forestall the rise of the problem of like or dislike for his patients in the mind of the psychiatrist. As he learns about the historical data which are responsible for the characterological development and for the psychopathology of the patient, the temptation of moral evaluation with the implication of acceptance or nonacceptance will be replaced by genetic understanding and therapeutic curiosity.

If a therapist feels that he likes or dislikes a patient who is under treatment, the reasons, as a rule, are not due to the patient's type of personality per se. The psychiatrist may like patients who are making satisfactory progress in treatment; he may be grateful to them for making his professional life more meaningful by their beneficent responses to his therapeutic endeavor. He may also like them because they augment his self-appreciation and his prestige. He may dislike a patient whose treatment has become stagnant; this may express doubts of his skill on the part of these patients. He may also dislike them because they may instil a feeling of skepticism regarding the purposefulness of his professional life. An even more significant possible cause for psychiatrists' dislike of patients stems from these patients' ability to touch off the psychiatrists' own unresolved anxieties. These, in turn, are frequently a measuring rod for these patients' anxiety and therefore a diagnostically and therapeutically valid tool in the hands of an alert psychiatrist.

These statements are not identical with the suggestion that every therapist should expect to be capable of treating persons suffering from any type of personality disorder. The contrary is true. In the course of his psychiatric career and with the aid of his supervised psychotherapeutic work, the therapist should learn to find out what type of patients respond best to his personality as it colors his type of therapeutic approach.* Of course, there are no rules of unfailing psychiatric validity to guide therapists in the difficult selection of suitable patients.

Here are a few examples taken from a host of similar ones, merely offered as signposts for a general orientation. A markedly schizoid psychiatrist may have a difficult and unsuccessful time with patients suffering from marked manic and depressive mood swings, and vice versa. A very maternal psychiatrist may needlessly get under the skin of an aloof patient who struggles for independence from a mother's domineering overprotection. Psychiatrists who like to reap the harvest of their collaborative therapeutic endeavor with patients in a not too distant future will work better with neurotics. For physicians whose psychiatric attention is more focused upon timeless therapeutic curiosity and research interest, work

---

* The young psychiatrist in psychoanalytic training is required to spend at least two hundred hours in supervisory discussions of several of his patients with experienced colleagues and to participate in several terms of clinical conferences.

with psychotics will be more rewarding. Anxious or forbidding personalities may not be helpful to patients suffering from anxiety states. Psychiatrists with markedly ingratiating or propitiating needs had best refrain from working with the suspicious paranoid patients. In the following chapter some further expedient criteria will be offered in this connection.

In now concluding the discussion of the role of the psychiatrist in the psychotherapeutic doctor-patient relationship, I wish to summarize my suggestions as follows:

It has been stated that the psychiatrist is expected to be stable and secure enough to be consistently aware of and in control of what he conveys to his patients in words and mindful of what he may convey by empathy. Also his need for operations aimed at his own security and satisfaction should not interfere with his ability to listen consistently to patients, with full alertness to their communications per se and, if possible, to the unworded implications of their verbalized communications. And the psychiatrist should never feel called upon to be anything more or less than the participant observer of the emotional experiences which are conveyed to him by his patients.

On the surface, these rules may seem obvious and easy to follow; yet they are not. As a matter of fact, they are offered to show the ideal goal for which the psychiatrist should strive. In actuality, none of us will consistently be able to live up to all of them. We have to bear in mind that no amount of inner security and self-respect protects the psychiatrist from being as much a subject of and vulnerable to the inevitable vicissitudes of life as is everyone else. This being the case, it is equally obvious that it may be difficult at times for each psychiatrist to maintain the role of the detached and alert participant observer of his patient. Indeed, special personal training is required before one can make a successful attempt at accomplishing this goal. The personal psychoanalysis which, for training purposes, has been repeatedly recommended in these pages as a requirement for the person who wishes to do intensive psychotherapy must also be recommended for reasons of the psychiatrist's personal development. It will help him to become sufficiently aware of his own problems and enable him to handle his interpersonal relationships at large, and therefore his professional relationships with his patients in particular, so that the first will not interfere with the latter. His personal analysis will serve as a valid means of acquainting him with the dynamic significance of his own early developmental history and his early patterns in interpersonal relationships as influential factors of his personality structure. This will bring about change in his personal adjustment if needed and hence improve his ability to keep the vicissitudes of his personal life apart from his professional life. It will also increase his skill in helping patients to reveal dissociated and repressed elements of their history and to recognize transference or parataxic factors in their present interpersonal experience with the therapist and others. The psychiatrist's own analysis, however, may not permanently protect him from being subject to more or less marked emotional reactions to the vicissitudes of the intercurrent events of his own life. These may interfere with the equanimity and serenity which are desirable features in the psychiatrist's professional dealings with his patients. Moreover, it is a difficult task to maintain the personal and the professional requirements for the psychiatrist as outlined, in the presence of the exacting emotional demands implied. Because of these two factors, repeated psychoanalytic inventories are recommended to psychiatrists throughout the course of their professional lives. And so it is that, because of the interrelatedness between the psychiatrist's and the patient's interpersonal processes and because of the interpersonal character of the psychotherapeutic process itself, any attempt at intensive psychotherapy is fraught with danger, hence unacceptable, where not preceded by the future psychiatrist's personal analysis.

# PART II

# THE PSYCHOTHERAPEUTIC PROCESS

## THE PATIENT AND THE THERAPIST

# CHAPTER V

## The Initial Interview

THE psychotherapeutic process begins with the first interview between the psychiatrist and a prospective patient. In order to start out right, the psychiatrist should remember that intensive psychotherapy is a mutual enterprise, if not a mutual adventure, between two people who are strangers and who are likely to be as different from each other as are the average personalities in this culture. Yet, at the same time, there is much more likeness between themselves and their mental patients than some psychiatrists may wish to see. "We are all much more simply human than otherwise," as H. S. Sullivan puts it (147).

The first interview should begin with the patient being asked about his complaints and about the nature of his problems and his suffering, which made him or his relatives or friends decide to have the patient ask for the advice of a psychiatrist. This information about the nature of the ailment of the mental patient should include the difficulties of long standing, which, as a rule, have been suffered by anyone seeking the advice of a psychiatrist. Coupled with this, the acute distress which has precipitated the patient's decision to see a psychiatrist should be investigated. After that the psychiatrist wishes to clarify, as early as possible in his contact with his prospective patient, whether the patient has come on his own volition, whether he has been advised to come by friends or relatives, or whether he has been prodded into doing so against his own wishes. If the patient has come to see the psychiatrist upon the decision of others rather than his own, the psychiatrist should center his efforts in the beginning on helping the patient convert his friends' decision into his own. The patient should learn to gain insight into his needs for psychiatric help and seek advice in his own right. The therapeutic process should be an interpersonal experience between him and the psychiatrist. The therapist can be useful to the patient only if he succeeds in getting the patient interested in fighting for his well-being on his own behalf rather than to please any third person.

It is of paramount significance for the whole course of the future treatment to have its issues outlined as clearly as possible in the initial interviews. This outline will furnish a helpful frame of reference whenever there is a threat of beclouding the issues in the course of treatment. The initial discussion should include the patient's presenting problems, a brief explanation of the philosophy, method, and aim of the treatment, and the establishment of the professional relationship between the psychiatrist and the prospective patient. This should be followed by a tentative appraisal of the duration of the treatment and by a tentative evaluation of possible changes for better or worse in the course of the treatment, including the sometimes inevitable temporary relapses.

I would like to repeat at this point what has been said by implication in the first chapter with regard to the doctor-patient relationship. I strongly advise against any attempt on the part of the psychiatrist to make things seemingly easier for the patient by pretending that the professional doctor-patient relationship is a social one. Deep down in his mind, no patient wants a nonprofessional relationship with his therapist, regardless of the fact that he may express himself to the contrary. Something in him senses, as a rule in spite of himself, that an extra-professional relationship with his psychiatrist will interfere with a patient's tendency toward change and improvement in his mental condition. Moreover, the psychiatrist who enters into a social relationship with his patient may easily become sufficiently involved himself in the nonprofessional aspects of this relationship to be rendered incapable of keeping control over the professional aspects of the doctor-patient relationship. Even assuming that the psychiatrist is a detached superman, who can keep the two sides of his relationship with the patient constructively apart, it is still advisable to avoid the necessity of having to do so. Even in pure culture, the business of psychotherapy and the handling of the professional doctor-patient relationship are complex and pregnant with difficulties and problems. Why complicate it by an additional problem which can be avoided? For all these reasons, I consider it the task of the psychiatrist to build up—

without unnecessary verbalization—the professional doctor-patient relationship of the type outlined in the first chapter, from the very beginning of his contact with a patient.

In that connection I remember with grief a schizophrenic woman whose reasonably good therapeutic prospects I damaged. Enticed by the utter skepticism and diffidence of the patient and of all her relatives regarding intensive psychothcrapy, I thought at the time it might be best in her case to start treatment with noncommittal talks and in a social setting. In spite of things going reasonably well, as we finally entered into a real professional treatment situation, and in spite of the establishment of a promising doctor-patient relationship, the patient irretrievably lost interest in the continuation of our efforts during one of her relapses. The family did likewise, the patient was taken to a state hospital against advice and has remained there since as a chronic incurable. It is my firm belief that this unhappy outcome could have been avoided, had the therapeutic situation been adequately clarified at the start of the treatment.

On the other hand, I remember with gratification the successful treatment of a catatonic girl. Before I started seeing her, she had been hospitalized for four years without any expectation for her final recovery. The goals and content of the therapeutic procedure and the necessity of excluding the intervention of any third person were clearly defined at the beginning of the treatment and were accepted with insight by the patient. An initial consensus between patient and psychiatrist about the nature of their collaborative professional relationship was established by implication. I consider it most likely that this fact was among the reasons responsible for the patient's ultimate recovery.* The suggestion of predicting the possibility of relapses does not presuppose my tacit agreement with those psychiatrists who consider relapses to be phenomena which inevitably precede any recovery from mental disorder. Many serious therapeutogenic relapses are due to lack of psychotherapeutic skill; the establishment of the doctrine of their necessity is often enough a poor rationalization for shortcomings in therapeutic knowledge, technique, or skill.

Some readers may consider the suggestion altogether redundant

* For a detailed report of this initial interview see Ref. 70.

that the patient be first encouraged to talk about his complaints in the initial interview. They may ask: What else should an initial conversation between a physician and a patient who seeks help start with but an account of his worries? At the present state of psychotherapeutic developments there is a need for making this apparently obvious statement. Psychoanalytic psychiatrists have been rightly trained, with great emphasis, to understand the emotional difficulties of their mental patients in terms of their early history and to make their patients view their problems in this light. This has been misinterpreted by many of them to mean that the historical causes for a patient's ailments should be investigated before seeking information as to the nature of the ailment itself. It will not make sense to any patient and should not make sense to any psychiatrist to inquire about the patient's past history before he has listened to the complaints which are responsible for the patient's seeking psychiatric advice.

Once the psychiatrist has succeeded in encouraging the patient's verbalization of his complaints and, if possible, in seeing the connection between his past and his present pains and difficulties, he still should not proceed to delve into the patient's childhood history. He should, first, be eager to collect information about the patient's present life and life-situation. He wants to know his age, his social and economic status and family background, the present family constellation, marital status, children, etc. Only by obtaining at least some rough data about the patient's actual life-circumstances, which furnish the background for his difficulties, can the psychiatrist adequately evaluate them and so form a reasonable judgment regarding diagnosis and prognosis.

In order to make this possible, the psychiatrist must set aside plenty of time for an initial interview. He cannot take care of the responsibility of deciding the future course of events in another human being's life and the possibilities of bringing forth changes in another person's life if he is pressed for time. I agree, moreover, with H. S. Sullivan, who suggests having any initial psychiatric interview interrupted by an interval which provides the opportunity for pondering about further information which the psychiatrist may wish to obtain and which the patient may wish to give. If that is not feasible, it may be wise to arrange for a second interview before any definite judgment is formed and before any statements as to the patient's condition and suggestions regarding therapeutic procedures are made. In the case of a prospective patient who is mute or out of contact, informative data should be obtained from relatives or friends and by the doctor who referred him.

How does the psychiatrist form an opinion regarding a prospective patient's condition and treatment necessities during and after the initial interviews, and how does he introduce concepts and methods of intensive psychotherapy to the patient? In answer to the first question: While consulting with the patient, the psychiatrist should, of course, not only listen to what the patient has to say but also pay attention to the way in which information is given. Does the prospective patient, for instance, show despair or apathy? Does he speak diffidently? Does he display discomfort, fear or anxiety, unhappiness or grief, etc.? Such observations will help the psychiatrist in his evaluation of the patient's actual feelings. They will also allow conclusions about the impression the patient wishes to make on the psychiatrist and, to a certain degree, regarding the expectations the patient has about the thoughts and feelings of the psychiatrist. This, in turn, will contribute to the therapist's understanding of the patient's personality.

Special attention should be paid to the way in which the patient behaves as he first enters the psychiatrist's office. Does he appear to be anxious or awkward, self-conscious, tearful, or shaky? Does he have difficulties in orienting himself? Does he behave as if in a daze? Does he appear to be in control of the situation? Is there a display of real or pretended self-reliance, a wish or a need to impress?

Another source of information comes from observing the patient's gait and posture, general appearance, facial expression, type of clothes and grooming, inadvertent motions. Observation of the appearance and behavior of the person accompanying the patient to his first interview (husband, wife, parent, friend) may furnish another source of helpful, collateral information. Also, attention should be paid to the patient's noticing or not noticing the surroundings and with what type of reaction he makes this evident. All these observations should be made as inconspicuously as possible, of course, in order to avoid any unnecessary addition to the self-consciousness. Great attention should also be paid to changes in mood which the patient may show during the interview and to changes in physical condition which the psychiatrist may observe or which the patient may mention. The patient should be encouraged to describe them in a detailed way, and he should be questioned as to their nature, their timing, and, if possible, their causes.

Some further clues to the patient's personality and about his condition may be obtained as the psychiatrist observes the patient's nonverbalized reactions to his questions or comments. He should note whether the patient's answers are to the point or whether they are not related to the contents of the psychiatrist's questions; whether the patient answers in the spirit of real or pretended self-reliance, security, insolence, etc.; whether he is pleasant or unpleasant; whether he shows surprise, distress, worry, anxiety, or a colorless or blank facial expression.

The questions which the psychiatrist asks the patient in order to try to get the information needed should not be formulated in such a way that they can be answered by saying only "Yes" or "No." Questions should be restrained, concrete, and simply meaningful. Many things are too complex for interrogation to be helpful at the time of the initial contact of the psychiatrist with the patient. If, for instance, a patient complains about homosexual tendencies, it is unwise in an initial interview to delve into an inquiry about the possible causes. Instead of asking the patient whether he considers his fear of women, perhaps his self-reflected engulfment or his unresolved overattachment to his mother, etc., responsible for his homosexuality, the psychiatrist should only ask the patient why he complains about it and why he wishes to get rid of it, if he does. The alleged truth of the afore-mentioned questions has nothing to do with the practical suggestion of not asking these questions at that time.

As the psychiatrist asks informative questions of the patient, he should recognize the patient's difficulties in answering them and should inexorably cut out purposeful attempts of some patients to evade correct answers by irrelevancies, preachments, or recitals. No one coming to an expert for help should be expected to be resentful of measured discipline in guidance or of prohibitive suggestions with regard to their interpersonal exchange, as long as this is done on the basis of the therapist's professional knowledge and authority and not on the basis of the irrational authority of the superior "healthy" doctor versus his "sick" patient. To repeat in this connection what has been emphasized before in a different context and with different wording: any humiliation of the patient should at all times be avoided, as in any interpersonal relationship. With mental patients it is of paramount importance because of their impaired self-esteem.

Once the psychiatrist has carefully collected and mulled over the information obtained from the patient and from his own observations, he should use his general life-experience and his professional experiences in evaluating these data. With these two bodies of knowledge in mind, certain conclusions can be derived from the data. Certain events may be presumed to have occurred according to the data collected, others cannot have occurred, both irrespective of the patient's own evaluation of his data.

Life-experience should enable the psychiatrist to differentiate between those aspects of the patient's communications which are characteristic of his educational or his cultural background and those which are effected by his emotional difficulties. An educated patient, for example, who speaks slowly may do so because of his temperament or because of neurotic inhibitions. An uneducated person may speak equally slowly because of his difficulties in expressing himself. A well-educated person may express himself very easily and skilfully, and his quick communication may be due to his educational training in the use of language. An uneducated person who speaks very easily and quickly may do so because of a psychopathological, for instance, a hypomanic state of outgoing mood.

In evaluating the contents of patients' communications, the psychiatrist must consider with equal care the colloquialisms and slang expressions, the use of which may frequently be conditioned by differences in patients' cultural and social backgrounds.

In the case of a foreigner it may happen that he uses the wrong words because of a lack of command of the language, which, if used by an American-born patient, might permit psychological conclusions regarding his state of mind. In the instance of a foreigner who uses the word "homely" when meaning to express appreciation for a "homelike" environment, this slip may be attributed to his unfamiliarity with the language. If an American-born person makes such an error, it may be assumed that it is due to a hostile impulse.

Serious errors along this line may occur if foreign-trained psychiatrists fail to keep in mind the difference in cultural backgrounds between their patients and themselves, before evaluating the observations gleaned from their patients. Such was an experience of mine, when I first came to this country. A patient told me about the troublesome aspects of her life which most justifiably lent themselves to a severe expression of grief and crying, especially as she discovered new, worrisome viewpoints while relating her story. Upon finishing her report, she immediately pulled herself together, opened her handbag, took out lipstick, rouge, and powder, and proceeded to put on fresh makeup with great care and utter disregard of the presence of the psychiatrist. My initial reaction was that here was serious pathological defiance toward the psychiatrist, or perhaps evidence of the patient's futile attempt to undo the effects of having legitimately broken down in a psychiatric interview. If so, it would lend itself to the interpretation of being due to severe anxiety at the full realization of her problems in the presence of another person. An American psychiatrist would immediately have recognized in this procedure the pattern of this culture.

Life-experience should also enable the psychiatrist to conclude from the data obtained from a patient that certain events which the patient does not mention must have occurred just the same, whereas other faithfully reported events cannot have taken place. For instance, if a patient reports that she is one partner in a happy homosexual relationship and that, preceding the homosexual entanglement, her marriage of many years' duration was a most successful one, the psychiatrist will immediately know that this cannot be so. If the homosexual experience is a genuinely happy one, then the marital one has not been, and vice versa.

In stating this, I do not mean to suggest that the psychiatrist convey his opinion to the prospective patient at the time. He may deem it best to make a mental note of it for future reference or to register some doubt which may or may not be taken in by the patient. Some remark such as "Is that so?" softly interjected, may serve the purpose.

Again, a person who appears to be very insolent may tell the psychiatrist about his wonderful childhood and the great amount of freedom he was granted. The psychiatrist will know that a happy childhood and the enjoyment of great freedom do not, as a general thing, produce an insolent individual. As a rule, impudence is a mask for deep-rooted insecurity. The "freedom" which an insolent and impudent person has allegedly enjoyed in his childhood has either been due to negligence on the part of the significant adults, which caused the child to feel worthless or hated, or been due to lack of advice offered to him in the early years when it is needed and when its absence makes the child feel insecure. A person who felt worthless and hated in his childhood may more or less purposely behave in an offensive way in later years, namely, insolently, in order to arouse hatred for his behavior. It is more bearable to feel hated for what one *does* than for what one *is*.

Much in the same way as these *exclusions*, certain *conclusions* can be made by the experienced psychiatrist, from the patient's data, irrespective of the patient's own awareness of them. A patient may complain about his general unhappiness in life and his failure in marriage. He may then remark that the only asset of his life is his love for his daughter, subsequently commenting upon how much his daughter resembles his sister-in-law. The conclusion the psychiatrist will draw from this report will quite naturally be that one of the causes for the patient's marital unhappiness is due to his attachment to his sister-in-law.*

In the same way, the professional experience of a psychiatrist may be helpful in precluding certain events and in concluding the probability of the existence of others. An example illustrating this is the case of a person who obviously is suffering from schizophrenia. He may tell the psychiatrist about his happy and harmonious infancy and childhood and about the unambiguous loving care given to him by his mother. Or a patient whose history and symptomatology show that he is suffering from marked manic-depressive mood swings may speak of the consistent guidance he

* Rogers gives several viewpoints similar to these and others suggested in this book, even though in a different frame of reference, in his *Counseling and Psychotherapy* (134).

was given by one significant adult or of the happy group integration which his family has accomplished.

The psychiatrist will know that a patient who is suffering from schizophrenia cannot have had a happy childhood history such as was given by the first patient and that a person who shows manic and depressive swings has, as a rule, been brought up under the shadow of great inconsistency in guidance by multiple parental figures, in an isolated group (71).

If it is true that the psychiatrist understands many implications in the communications of the patient of which the patient himself is not aware, the question is in order as to what it is that interferes with the patient's awareness of what seems to be so evident to his listener. With regard to childhood experiences of which the patient is lacking in awareness, it may be due, first, to the general normal amnesia which human beings develop for early childhood experiences (74, 137). A second reason may be that some unhappy people wish to glorify their past in an attempt to compensate for their present suffering. A third group of people may try to forget the hardships which their parents inflicted upon them in their childhood because they do not wish to blame them or to bear a grudge against them, for fear of breaking the Fifth Commandment. Also their own low self-respect may call forth the need to maintain the pretense of great respect for their parents which they do not feel for themselves.

The myth of the happiness of childhood years which is maintained as a general comforting concept in this culture facilitates the patient's faculty of forgetting his childhood hardship, since patients are just as dependent on current concepts in public opinion as are their "healthy" fellow-men. This myth has remained powerful in the thinking of people of this culture, in spite of the results of Freud's scrutiny of people's childhood experiences, which showed only too frequently warp and frustration.

One more reason for the dissociation of childhood memories seems to stem from the fact that many frustrated, thwarted, unhappy parents compensate for the hardship of their own lives and the people who caused it by maltreating their young children, the only persons whom they can mistreat with impunity. If they deny the recall of unhappy aspects of infancy and childhood, it may mean (to them) that they were not unhappy and also that they did not make their children unhappy.

It appears then that life offers little happiness to all too many adults; hence they may maintain the religious concept of future happiness in the hereafter, or they cling to the myth of past happiness in their childhood. In order to do the latter effectively, solid processes of dissociation or repression have to be activated. It requires the help of another person, the psychiatrist, who, in his turn, has come to grips with his own childhood memories, to bring them to recall.

Another basic cause for the universal difficulty of lifting childhood amnesias stems from the fact that one can remember events only in the "modality in which they appear first," as Goldstein put it. He goes on to say that "remembrance . . . presupposes a similarity between the situation in which the organism was at the time of the experience" (74). This presupposition, of course, does not hold for the recall of childhood memories later in life. Adult experiences are all too highly "schematized" and "conventionalized" as compared with the genuine "freshness, spontaneity, and originality of early experience and memory" (cf. Schachtel, Ref. 137).

Under the specific conditions of the psychotherapeutic situation, at least part of this schematization and conventionalization of human existence and experience is undone. Therefore, events and certainly some emotional reflections of events which otherwise cannot be remembered may be subject to recall under psychotherapeutic guidance. Technical suggestions about this part of the psychotherapeutic procedure with regard to lost memories in childhood and later and the reasons for the loss of recall of experiences in later life will be discussed in connection with the problems of interpretation (Part II, pp. 80–84).

As to the question of what type of person is eligible and should be advised to undertake psychoanalytic psychotherapy, my answer would be: anyone who consults a psychiatrist about marked emotional difficulties in living of which he wishes to be freed and who appears to be flexible and sincere, or shows the potentialities for both. By this I mean all types of character neuroses, neurotics, and, according to recent experience, also psychotics. People who show symptoms indicative of marked organic damage to the brain (arteriosclerotics, seniles, paretics) are excluded. This does not mean to say that these people may not get relief from intensive psychotherapy but that, in all probability, no marked personality changes will be accomplished. The people who suffer from psychosomatic symptoms, the emotional roots of which can be brought home to them, constitute another eligible group.

A high I.Q. is not a prerequisite for undergoing psychoanalysis. This holds all the more true, since, of course, there are many persons whose intellectual abilities are curtailed because of emotional conditions which may be favorably influenced by psychoanalytic psychotherapy. A good innate intelligence may help, though, in speeding the procedure.

As to the age of the persons who should undertake psychoanalytic psychotherapy: before accepting children and other young people for intensive treatment, an attempt should be made to improve the youngsters' emotional difficulties in living by treating the significant adult or adults who seem to be responsible for the condition of the young person. Frequently the children do not need treatment when the responsible adults are reached successfully. In all cases the parents or one parent should be seen and, if possible, psychoanalytically indoctrinated simultaneously with their child's treatment (35, 87, 132).*

Regarding the older-aged groups, psychiatrists used to think that women past the middle of their thirties and men past the middle of their forties were no longer flexible enough and had to work through too long a span of personal history to undertake psychoanalytic psychotherapy. Psychotherapeutic changes for these people were also considered to be not too favorable because sexual gratification was considered a *sine qua non* of a happy life-adjustment (cf. pp. 32–38). Recent experience has led most psychiatrists to change this viewpoint. It is true that there is a longer life-history to be considered, and there may be a somewhat lesser degree of personal flexibility in these people. However, these liabilities, as a rule, are amply made up for in those older persons who are eager to overcome their difficulties by a more eminent matureness, a larger body of life-experience, and, above all, by a greater sense of urgency in finding better ways of living for the shorter

* See also the literature on child analysis quoted in Ref. 34.

span of life left to them. I personally have been gratified by being instrumental in the accomplishment of marked improvements in living of three women patients and one man who started their treatments during the second part of their fifties, and four women patients and one man who started treatment during the second part of their forties.

In recent years psychological testing and graphology have been used successfully to help with the initial evaluation of the personality of the psychiatric patient and of his outlook (Rorschach, Szondi, Murray's Thematic Apperception Test) (126). Augusta Slesinger, of New York, has developed psychiatric techniques for approaching her patients which are designed to speed reaching emotional material which otherwise may remain out of awareness for a long time. Her method is designed to improve personality evaluation and therapy. She asks patients to close their eyes and to pay attention and associate to entoptic images; or she requests that they try to visualize inner pictures of themselves and give their revealing associations to these pictures. Another device which she uses is to ask patients startling questions such as: What would you do if you had all the money you wanted? The answers, which frequently are most surprising to the patients, serve as background for further psychoanalytic investigation. Slesinger's book on the subject is to be published soon.

After the psychiatrist has collected sufficient data to judge the patient's therapeutic needs, he should work toward establishing mutual understanding and validation of these needs. No doubt every human being has an innate tendency toward health, both mental and physical, just as one has a tendency toward fluid intake when thirsty and toward the intake of food when hungry (70, 147). This does not mean, however, that the conscious wish for health can be equally taken for granted. There are too many interferences with the tendency toward health in a person's inner organization and life. It is for this reason that the psychiatrist must ascertain whether or not the patient actually wishes treatment and change. Where such wishes do not exist, the first therapeutic step should be toward their encouragement.

Once the patient's own wish for treatment and recovery has been established or its future development may be anticipated with reasonable certainty, the attempt should then be made to establish a consensus between patient and therapist about the following problems: What are the problems, difficulties, and suggestions for which the patient seeks solution and help? It has proved to be most helpful if and when patient and therapist can agree about at least one primary problem in the patient's living which needs therapeutic consideration. Frequently this will not be possible. But at least an attempt should be made in that direction. After that, the philosophy and method of intensive psychotherapy must be briefly introduced to the understanding of the prospective patient. The way to go about this will depend upon the patient's degree of disturbance, his general educational background, and his knowledge of psychiatric, psychological, and psychoanalytic concepts. The direction of these explanations should be along the following lines: the patient would not be disturbed and would not come to a psychiatrist for help or advice if it were not for the fact that he did not understand his presenting symptoms or the reasons and dynamics behind his anxiety. It may be explained to the patient that this lack of understanding is due to the fact that important emotional experiences from which the patient's difficulties spring, in part, have been "forgotten," are not available for recall. The patient should then be told that this fact is among the reasons for his not knowing how to cope with his emotional difficulties, so that his private fight against his misery has been destined to failure.

Psychosomatic complaints with whose psychogenic nature the patient is familiar may be explained as a sign of pressing emotional problems which are totally or in part barred from the patient's awareness. In the case of an uninitiated patient who does not realize the psychogenic nature of his physical symptomatology, such explanations have to be postponed, of course. They would lend themselves to the rise of the impression in the patient's mind that the doctor does not take his complaints seriously or that he considers them to be the result of mere imagination.

It may, furthermore, be explained to the prospective patient that the therapeutic process is aimed at bringing a sufficient amount of dissociated material into awareness so that understanding of it may follow. Then it can be explained that this goal may be accomplished by the psychiatrist helping patients to verbalize and formulate their experiences in his presence. The idea should then be introduced to the patient that his ever growing awareness and understanding of the contents, history, and dynamics of his interpersonal processes are geared to enable him to understand and to cope efficiently with the troublesome aspects of his life or even to eliminate them, outer circumstances permitting. He should, furthermore, learn to understand that his immediate complaints and symptoms are mutually interlocked with his problems and difficulties and therefore are expected to yield in the course of this psychotherapeutic process. Finally, it should be made clear to the patient that this is possible only if he and the psychiatrist undertake a thorough scrutiny of his life-history and especially of the history of his interpersonal relationships and their reflection on the doctor-patient relationship.

Explanations of this or a similar type, of course, can be given only to people whose mental disturbance is not so grave that it bars verbalized communication or that it greatly reduces the patient's ability to listen. To the more seriously disturbed person, one may not be able to say much more than something on the order of: "There must be reasons for your feeling so bad or for your not getting along or for your not being interested in this business of living, about which you do not know, nor does the psychiatrist know about them offhand. Let us try to investigate them with each other."

In the case of a mute patient, who gives no indication of whether or not he has heard the psychiatrist, the initiation into treatment may have to be done through occasional remarks regarding the patient's history and difficulties and by connecting those as the occasion arises with bits of information about psychotherapeutic perspectives. In order to do this successfully, the psychiatrist may have to use the data he obtains from patients' relatives (see section on "Contacts with Relatives," pp. 214–24).

Sometimes an inarticulate patient gives the psychiatrist an opening, making it possible for him to interject one or another initiating remark, as in the following example: A patient was sitting naked on the floor when the psychiatrist first saw him. He greeted the doctor by asking, "Can you tell me what it is that makes me behave like an animal?" This gave the psychiatrist the opportunity to offer the suggestion that the patient had taken, as it were, a leave of absence from his human existence in order to gain time for rest and relaxation. Seeing that the patient had accepted this suggestion, the psychiatrist went on to explain that this rest period could also be used for the integration of the painful experience to which the patient had been exposed before he withdrew into the animal-like form of existence. This could best be done by a collaborative investigation of the known and unknown facts which had led up to the unbearable previous hurts in the patient's life. Thus the first step was taken toward explaining the philosophy and method of psychotherapy to a psychotic patient.*

Another seriously disturbed and, as a rule, rather inarticulate patient shouted at the psychiatrist who tried to arouse the wish for recovery in her, "Don't you realize that I am not a bit interested?" The psychiatrist's reply was that she was fully aware of the patient's present lack of interest in her recovery and in any procedure which was aimed at it. Therefore, she suggested that the patient operate for the time being "on borrowed belief," that is, that she follow the therapist's belief in the possibly favorable results of their joint scrutiny of the dissociated experiences responsible for the patient's lack of interest in and of hope for a better way of living.

The psychiatrist, of course, will be called upon to tell a patient or his relatives, if the patient is too disturbed to communicate with him, about the opinion he has formed regarding the patient's condition and need for treatment. He may be inclined to encourage the patient or his relatives by depicting the situation and the treatment procedures less seriously than, in his own judgment, he really believes them to be. He will not be doing them a favor by any such misrepresentation. By and large, people who come to see a psychiatrist these days do so because of acute suffering and serious predicament. They feel encouraged if the psychiatrist realizes the severity of their difficulties and does not minimize them.

The same holds true with regard to the inclination of some psychiatrists to impress their prospective patients with a quick diagnosis or prognosis which they sometimes even venture to give over the telephone, when a patient asks for an interview. Such proce-

* For further information about all questions of psychoanalytic technique as mentioned here and later see Refs. 31, 72, 99, and literature cited there.

dure cannot be counteradvised too strenuously. First of all, there are only a few cases in which even the most experienced psychiatrist is capable of forming a diagnostic opinion solely by virtue of a contact over the telephone. Furthermore, if the psychiatrist is not acquainted with the person who asks for an interview by telephone, he cannot evaluate the effect of his diagnosis upon the person at the other end of the wire. He may harm the person seriously by diagnosing him at random, and he may curtail his own later judgment by preconceived diagnostic conceptions. Moreover, far from being impressed by such alacrity, the patient, as a rule, will resent it as being indicative of the psychiatrist's lack of appreciation for the complexities involved.

At the present developmental state of psychotherapy, it is frequently wise also to refrain from well-founded diagnostic statements even in personal interviews. I am thinking especially of the diagnosis of schizophrenia as being connected in the minds of many lay people and unfortunately also in the judgment of many psychiatrists with the connotation of psychotherapeutic inaccessibility. They believe that only shock treatments and psychosurgery can help to relieve the suffering of these patients, even though they realize that this may be accomplished at the expense of the emotional integrity and further development of the patients' personalities. The diagnosis "schizophrenia" given by a psychiatrist of my school of psychiatric thinking is coupled with the knowledge that he and the patient are heading for hard work, but it is by no means offered in the spirit of prognostic discouragement. But this diagnosis may be devastatingly discouraging to the semieducated patient or relative, who has heard that schizophrenics cannot be treated by psychotherapy.

Moreover, the old psychiatric diagnostic terminology which is built up in terms of curable and noncurable psychopathological entities is bound to be revised in the light of recent psychiatric progress in psychotherapeutic understanding, skill, and knowledge. Since a new classification has not as yet been accomplished, diagnosing of mental disorder is misleading for the time being, especially in a therapeutic frame of reference.* I, for one, have made it a rule during the past few years to explain these facts to patients

* At present, efforts to work out a new classification are under way under the auspices of the American Psychiatric Association.

and relatives when they press me for a diagnosis, so that they may understand that my refusal to give it is not a deceptive evasion.

The explanation of the psychotherapeutic process should be followed by a short discussion of expectations about the outcome of the treatment. The ideal goals of psychotherapy and the practical expectation to be derived from it were given in the preceding chapter, where they were discussed for the benefit of the psychiatrist. Abbreviated variations of what was said there about the goal and expectation of psychotherapy may be used in the psychiatrist's discussion of this topic with the prospective patient and/or his relatives, toward the end of the initial interview (see also the section on "Termination of Treatment," pp. 188–94).

When methods of and outlook for therapy have been discussed, the matter of practical decisions and prospects of treatment must be considered. They have to be taken up in detail with the patient himself or, in the case of a psychotic who cannot be contacted, with his relatives. The discussion should include the choice of the psychiatrist, the question as to whether the patient should remain ambulatory or be hospitalized, a tentative approximation of the time needed, the number of weekly interviews, and the question of fees.

The choice of psychiatrist should be considered from the viewpoint of the personal suitability of the therapist to the needs of that particular patient. At the turn of the century, when Sigmund Freud first developed a teachable method and technique of doing psychotherapy, psychoanalysts were inclined to think that the psychotherapeutic tools were all that were needed, regardless of the type of personality. At that time it was thought that any psychiatrist who was emotionally stable, was well trained in the use of psychotherapeutic tools, and showed integrity and medical responsibility could treat any type of patient. We know now that the success or failure of psychoanalytic psychotherapy is, in addition, greatly dependent upon the question of whether or not there is an empathic quality between the psychiatrist and the patient. A careful evaluation regarding the personalities of both patient and doctor and of the psychopathology of the patient should be helpful in the decision. The problems of psychopathology and character structure of patient and doctor, which were previously discussed, should, of course, be included. In this vein, the therapist who has conducted the initial interviews for purposes of consultation must ask himself whether or not he feels equal to treating that particular patient. Also, he must ask the patient whether or not the latter feels the desire for treatment by the consultant. Further discussion about the choice of the prospective analyst should include a consideration of the sex and, in the present cultural era of unfortunate prejudices, of the prospective therapist's race or religion. The patient's initial response to this question will almost always be in the affirmative, for various reasons. In the first place, the average mental patient will be fearful of hurting the doctor's feelings by giving a negative answer; second, he will be inclined to act upon the recommendation of the person who sent him to this particular psychiatrist; and, last but not least, he will be fearful of having to make another new contact and another new decision. In the presence of these facts, the psychiatrist should not allow his judgment to be influenced by being flattered by the patient's affirmative answer. He should keep in mind that, other things being equal, the patient's decision would have been in favor of any colleague who happened to be the first one consulted.

The decision about ambulatory treatment or hospitalization in borderline states must be influenced by the following considerations. The decision should not be made in the false spirit of maintaining the patient's "freedom" at all costs. What means "freedom" to a person who is mentally stable may mean nothing but an unbearable, compulsory burden to the mentally incapacitated, who cannot live up to the standards and expectations of their environment (70). There are patients, however, for whom hospitalization adds in large measure to the initial hurt of being afflicted with a mental disorder. The psychiatrist may not be able to dispose of this prejudice immediately. In these cases the psychiatrist should avoid hospitalization if he possibly can. He may be rewarded for the increase in responsibility and actual work which he incurs, because he may forego changes for the worse and an unnecessary prolongation of the treatment period (69).

A third group of patients urge hospitalization without having their condition warrant it. They are the people who long for temporary riddance of their responsibilities or for dependence, with the dubious privilege of being taken care of by others. The psychiatrist should decide carefully, in each particular case, which procedure will be more important and therapeutically more valid: the relief or the added scar of temporary hospitalization for the seriously ill, and the therapeutically valid relief or the pampering effect in the case of the milder forms of disorder. The reluctance of the therapist to assume personally the responsibility for the ambulatory treatment of a patient, who may or may not have to be hospitalized at some time during the course of the treatment, ought not to be a consideration influencing his decision. Neither should the psychiatrist be reckless in evaluating both sides of the picture for reasons of his personal ambition.

The approximate time required for treatment prior to the recovery of the patient is difficult to predict. At the present time attempts are made at various psychiatric centers to abbreviate the treatment period for psychiatric patients (5, 6, 118). This book deals with the treatment of patients for whom the goal of recovery is one with insight, versus social recovery (see Introduction, pp. ix–xv). This goal can be obtained at the present state of psychotherapeutic skill and knowledge only with long-term, intensive psychoanalytic psychotherapy. This refers to the more serious type of neuroses (obsessional and phobic states), many character analyses, and the psychoses. In some of these conditions the psychiatrist may be able to make a tentative prognostic prediction. It should be understood, though, that this prediction cannot be binding. With other patients the psychiatrist may suggest a trial period of treatment of from anywhere between six weeks to three or four months, after which time he may be better prepared to make a tentative prediction about the duration.

There are additional reasons for starting treatment with a trial period for the benefit of the patient and of the therapist. During this period the psychiatrist and the patient can check on the validity of the initial evaluation of the possibility of therapy and of a workable treatment situation between the two people concerned.

During the trial period, therapy should be conducted, in principle, the same way in which it will be done while the psychotherapeutic procedure is in progress. However, one should be cautious about delving too deeply into material which is fraught with intense anxiety. The release of too much anxiety is unwise, if not dangerous, until the therapist feels certain that through continuation of treatment he will be available to help the patient handle his anxiety.

After the therapist feels that he is ready for a tentative evaluation of the time required for a patient's treatment, he should keep in mind the following considerations when giving a time estimate to the patient or his relatives. On the one hand, he does not wish to frighten a patient who may not have heard previously about the attendant requirements of intensive psychotherapy by giving what may seem to such a patient an extravagant statement. On the other hand, he does not wish to make too much of an understatement about the possible duration of the treatment, misled by an erroneous concept of what may discourage a prospective patient. When it becomes evident that the psychiatrist's time estimate was too optimistic, without this possibility having been mentioned, the price which patient and therapist may have to pay is likely to be very high. Distrust and discouragement on the part of the patient may reach the point where they amount to a real threat to the future productive continuation of the therapeutic collaboration. Roughly speaking, the psychiatrist may give a tentative time estimate of not less than a year or two to patients suffering from neuroses, and two years or more to the more seriously disturbed people, the psychotics.

Regarding the frequency of psychotherapeutic interviews, psychoanalysts used to think that their patients should meet them for five or six interviews a week. Under the pressure of the shortage in psychiatric manpower before, during, and following the war, many psychiatrists began experimenting with a reduced number of interviews a week. As a result of this, many of them have found that such a reduction in the number of weekly interviews is not detrimental to the psychotherapeutic process. The positive and negative sides of the patient's attachment to and his dependence on the psychiatrist, in its real and in its parataxic aspects, may be less vigorous and complex. Hence it will be less difficult to resolve both attachment and dependence when there are fewer interviews.

With some types of patients, for instance, manic-depressive personalities, a reduced number of therapeutic hours seems to work even more successfully. Two or three interviews per week seem to be all that these people, who are untrained and not gifted in introspection, are able to handle advantageously (71); see also pp. 80–84. Treatment in terms of reduction in the number of hours per week does not mean that psychotherapy is less intensive. Reduction in intensity has to be safeguarded against by an increase of watchful alertness on the part of the psychiatrist. In my personal experience I have found that the psychotherapeutic progress of the average patient did not seem to be reduced by our meeting three times weekly in comparison to the previous schedule of five or six interviews weekly. With some difficult patients, I like to start at the rate of four hours per week, changing to three as soon as the psychotherapeutic process is well under way.

In some of the psychoanalytically oriented mental hygiene clinics, some patients can be seen only once a week, and even under this condition I have seen a number of encouraging results. As a rule, it worked out beneficially to prolong the duration of these weekly interviews to $1\frac{1}{2}$ hours as compared with the classical 50- to 60-minute interview. The demands on the receptiveness, alertness, and intentness of the psychiatrist who works with this type of schedule are very heavy, but the nature of his contribution may be quite rewarding.*

If possible, the therapist should not begin treatment with several new patients at the same time. It is advantageous to concentrate on becoming acquainted with one new person's basic data at a time without interference from the same demand regarding a second one. An interval of from two to four weeks between the start of psychotherapy with two new patients seems indicated. This may necessitate a delay in beginning treatment with a new patient with whom the therapist has reached a mutual agreement regarding their working with each other. If this should happen, it must be frankly discussed with the patient.

Before treatment actually begins, there should be a discussion and settlement of fees. This is more important than in the case of other medical specialties, because the patient or his relatives incur

* For training purposes it is strongly recommended that the young psychiatrist work on a schedule of three to five interviews weekly with several patients before he undertakes seeing patients for a lesser number of scheduled hours per week.

the obligation of a continuous expense over a long and uncertain period of time. The settlement of the fee should be determined by the following factors. Psychiatric services—that is, the attempt to help a person overcome his emotional difficulties in living—are priceless if successful or worthless if they fail. It is through these attempts, nevertheless, that the therapist makes his living, so that the settlement of his fees has to be determined by the market value of psychiatric services at a given time and in a given area. The degree in variation of these fees must be in proportion to the financial status of the patient and according to the number of patients whom the psychiatrist has accepted at both average and reduced fees at the time.

An initial understanding should be reached as to scheduled interviews missed by either doctor or patient. Interviews missed by the doctor should be rescheduled if important or if requested. This also holds true for interviews missed by the patient for valid reasons. It should be understood that, as a rule, patient and doctor should notify each other as far ahead as possible when scheduled interviews must be broken. A patient who breaks an appointment for valid reasons should not be charged, even if he is unable to give previous notice, as in emergencies such as acute illness, sudden death in the family, etc. If the patient repeatedly misses interviews for invalid reasons, warning should be given, and thereafter charges should be made. In some cases the doctor should consider discontinuation of treatment, since the patient's breaking appointments continuously may be indicative of his lack of interest in serious psychotherapeutic collaboration. Patients who cannot afford adequate payments for their treatment should be treated for nominal fees or without pay.* The old psychoanalytic concept that psychotherapy will not be successful with patients who do not make a financial sacrifice to obtain it, regardless of their economic status, is an unfortunate misconception engendered by misleading teachings of our modern culture. This does not mean to deny the desirability of nominal payments where possible,

* At present an increasing number of psychoanalytically oriented mental hygiene clinics operated by the communities and the Veterans Administration and of low-cost clinics operated by psychoanalytic training centers try to take care of the surplus number of patients without adequate means who cannot be handled in private practice.

for the sake of the maintenance of the self-respect of the patient who does not wish to obtain something for nothing. This statement, of course, does not refer to people who are treated under a health insurance plan or under similar arrangements. People who are financially capable of paying for the professional services they require should, quite naturally, be held responsible for doing so. In the case of young people below the age of full earning capacity, whose parents pay for their treatment, it frequently proves to be wise for them to pay part of the fees from their small income or allowance in order to emphasize that the treatment situation is actually their own and not their parents' concern and responsibility.

I have discussed the financial aspects of intensive psychotherapy extensively because the attitude toward money all too frequently constitutes one of the problems of the psychiatric patient in this culture. He should be free to discuss it openly and thoroughly against the background of a clarified attitude toward money matters on the part of his therapist personally and in their mutual relationship.

Some noted psychiatrists have advocated that interviews missed by the patient should be paid for, irrespective of frequency and validity of reasons. This has been explained on the basis of the fact that the doctor contracts for a certain part of his earning capacity in terms of time with the patient. This is indeed true. Yet I feel that it is not the psychiatrist's privilege to be exempt from the generally accepted custom of our culture in which one is not paid for services not rendered (see also Ref. 93). I realize, of course, that the unforeseen loss of income-producing time is a handicap. I do not see any way in which this can be avoided in the above-mentioned incidents without interfering with the self-respect of the psychiatrist and the dignity of the profession. Moreover, to a productive personality, such free time may be of the essence.

# CHAPTER VI

## Introductory Remarks on the Psychotherapeutic Procedure

A DEFINITION of the meaning and the goal of intensive psychotherapy has been given in the preceding chapters. The principles of psychotherapy have been discussed in terms of the requirements for the therapist and as they apply to the initial interview with the patient. I shall now discuss the psychotherapeutic procedure in its progression. As mentioned before, it begins the moment the psychiatrist and the prospective patient meet and establish a relationship for the purpose of determining the patient's difficulties and the means of alleviating them.

The functioning of the psychotherapeutic process is implemented by the mutual collaboration of psychiatrist and patient. As previously mentioned, the first psychotherapeutic tool used by the psychiatrist is listening intelligently to patients' communications, such as spontaneous complaints and reports about connecting factual and emotional biographical data, especially from childhood, and about recent and previous private interpersonal experiences, such as reveries, dreams, delusions, and hallucinations. Another integral part of the psychiatrist's task is to promote the production of patients' data by asking pertinent and simply meaningful informative questions; also one should encourage patients' associative thinking and production and their observation of and reports on marginal thoughts and physical sensations during the therapeutic interview. The therapist continues to utilize his tools by offering meaningful interpretations; by investigating patients' interpretive thinking through asking correct interpretive questions at the proper time; by tying together both with and for patients the seemingly disconnected pieces of information and insight gradually obtained with the help of the afore-mentioned procedures; by paying close attention to his own inner reactions to

[ 69 ]

patients' manifestations as an additional access to the understanding of their implicit meaning; and by guiding patients in repeatedly working through in various and sundry connections the emotional experiences which have come to their awareness and to their understanding.

The purpose of listening intelligently and of asking for pertinent information is, first, to encourage verbalization and formulation of all that patients know about the troublesome aspects of their lives and the connecting data and to facilitate recall of part of what seemed "forgotten"; second, to obtain and to convey to patients a valid picture of the nature of their difficulties and eventually of the structure of their personalities.

The purpose of interpretation and interpretive questions is to bring dissociated and repressed experiences and motivations to awareness and to show patients how, unknown to themselves, repressed and dissociated material finds its expression in and colors verbalized communications and behavior patterns such as their actions, attitudes, and gestures.

The most important psychotherapeutic material with which patients and psychiatrist must work stems from the vicissitudes of the doctor-patient relationship in its real and in its distorted aspects. This material includes positive and negative transference and parataxic distortions. It also includes security operations in relation to the therapist, as a conscious defense against psychotherapeutic procedures and unconscious "resistance" against the psychiatrist and the effectiveness of the psychotherapeutic process and the emotional reactions to the patient and to his productions on the part of the psychiatrist (30, 38, 72, 99).

# CHAPTER VII

## Associations, Marginal Thoughts, Physical Sensations, and Their Usage in Psychotherapy

### 1. ASSOCIATIONS

SUGGESTIONS have been given in the previous chapters about the modes of listening intelligently and eliciting information from the patient by pertinent, meaningful questions. Now I wish to discuss the use in the psychotherapeutic process of the next tool mentioned in the previous chapter: the encouragement of the patients' associations and the observation of marginal thoughts and physical sensations as sources of psychotherapeutically valid information.

"Free associations" are an integral part of the original concept of psychoanalytic therapy (30, 37, 72, 99). Pertinent to this concept, it should be made clear that the associative thinking of a patient is "free" only in the sense that he is encouraged to ventilate freely all thoughts, feelings, and fantasies as they occur during the psychoanalytic interview, without any conventional restrictions. As to their content, however, these associations are not free because they are co-determined in their contents by preceding and contemplated subsequent thoughts, feelings, and associations. C. G. Jung was the first to demonstrate this clearly in his experimental studies on associations. It may be more exactly said, therefore, that the analysts' request that patients express themselves without choice, purpose, guidance, or questions about everything as it comes to mind is an integral part of classical psychoanalysis. This was considered the most adequate way of bringing dissociated or repressed material to patients' awareness and of subsequently discussing with them its contents, dynamics, and genetics.*

* Repression and dissociation are the main processes used to bar outward events or inner thoughts and feelings from awareness and to prevent their recall into consciousness. Consequently, the terms "repression" and "dissocia-

At the present state of psychoanalytic knowledge about repressive and dissociative processes, it proves to be unnecessarily time-consuming, in my experience, to make the patient's free associations a central part of intensive psychotherapy. In borderline patients and with outright psychotics this procedure carries with it the possible danger of inducing and increasing disintegrated thinking. For this reason encouraging psychotic patients to freely associate is strictly contraindicated. This, of course, does not mean that the spontaneous associations of psychotics should be discouraged if at times that is all they can produce.

The conventional barriers to free communication with the psychiatrist were another reason for Freud's recommendation of the method. Meanwhile, the lifting of these barriers has been partly accomplished by Freud's own teachings and their influence upon changes in cultural patterns. Other sociologically determined changes in cultural evaluations of secretiveness about embarrassing unconventionalities, of course, have also contributed. In the early nineteen hundreds, when psychoanalytic therapy was first conceived, people did not speak so freely about material which was considered most "embarrassing," namely, sexual matters, as they do today. By and large, people now speak more easily about sexual matters than about the "embarrassing" topics of the present era, such as their feelings of hostility and tenderness (cf. pp. 80–84). This holds true to a certain extent with people in general and especially so in the dealings of mental patients with their psychiatrists. The latter situation is partly due to the present widespread knowledge of the requirements for psychoanalytic therapy. As a rule, therefore, such devices as the encouragement of free associations are now not indispensable as a tool for conquering the reluctance of patients to talk about unconventional material. If there is reluctance, the cause is frequently from totally different sources. These will be discussed in the sections on "Resistance" and "Intentional Blocking" (pp. 107–18 and 118–19). Free association not only fails to take care of these types of reluctance but also can easily be

---

tion" are used throughout this book to cover all operations which serve this purpose and are therefore subject to interpretive psychotherapy. For further mechanisms used in the service of the same or similar motivations see Refs. 36, 37, 54, 78a, 147.

misused in their service. Some corroboration of this may be found in statements volunteered by more than one former patient to the effect that they were intentionally able to exclude from communication certain associations about which they were hesitant to speak while they were allegedly employing free associations.

The second reason for a more restricted use of free association is a consequence of the shift in emphasis of the patients' productions. The interest of the psychoanalytic psychiatrist is now directed toward what motivates each patient to keep material in dissociation and toward the reactions of the patient in response to repressed material which mounts into awareness, rather than toward its contents per se.

As a result, the attention of the psychiatrist has recently been focused more upon the investigation of the ego-defenses, the security operations of patients as they are mobilized by the psychotherapeutic process, than upon the scrutiny of the contents of their dissociations and repressions. To repeat: free associations used to be a most helpful device for gaining access to patients' repressed and dissociated thoughts and feelings and to doctors' and patients' understanding of the meaning of their contents. At present they are less useful, however. To many of us uncovering the dynamics motivating these repressions and dissociations and investigating patients' security operations can be better accomplished, as a rule, by skilfully eliciting and listening alertly to the patient's directed and informative statements than by encouraging his free associations.

One danger implied in overrating the significance of free associations is the possibility that the therapist may fail to pay close enough attention to apparently inconsequential factual events in the current lives of patients. The search for historical material and for timeless interpersonal processes outside patients' awareness is certainly of the greatest importance for understanding the psychopathology of every mental disorder. But the investigation of a patient's current interpersonal dealings should never, under any circumstances, be neglected. It is mandatory for the psychiatrist to press for their recital because they are an important source of information for uncovering ego-defenses and security operations and the motivating anxiety behind them (see also the section on

"Dreams," pp. 161–73). More often than not, this material may be neglected if the psychiatrist is prone to leave the selection of topics for discussion too much to the discretion of patients.

That the small events of current everyday life are important in understanding the psychopathology of patients is well illustrated by the following experience. A patient evaded reporting current or past data of her daily life. Instead, she indulged in the production of never ending free associations of nondescript feelings and emotions. Urged to interrupt this stream of associations and to give some information about daily events, she began speaking of her daily life by offering self-derogatory remarks about her habit of always being late for appointments. The patient went on to say that she wondered why she so seldom was ready to leave home sufficiently early to enable her to be on time and that, despite being a quick dresser, she was always rushed and under pressure when getting ready to keep any appointment. Each time she was preparing to go out of the house, the closets and her bureau drawers had to be put in order before she left. If she simply didn't have time to straighten things and left some disorder, she felt uncomfortable most of the time she was out. This complaint seemed surprising because it came from a person who otherwise was remarkably free from obsessional symptoms. Finally, the patient spoke of her mother's emphatically impressing upon her that she should always keep the rooms and her personal things in order and not go out leaving disorder. An accident might befall the patient while out, or she might be taken ill at any time. In her absence people would see her disorderly home and judge her and her upbringing accordingly. After the recital of this recurrent episode in her daily life, the patient herself realized, for the first time, her dependence upon the approval and her fear of the disapproval of her mother, as well as of the anonymous people conjured up by her mother. Subsequently she was able to face the connecting feelings of mild anxiety which were constantly shadowing her life. The patient recognized her rambling on about nondescript feelings as her weapon against evidencing her sense of anxiety.

Another example is offered in the treatment history of an obsessional patient who, time and again, complained about the course of her analytic work because the psychiatrist constantly pressed

her to report the routine events of the preceding day, no matter
how inconsequential they seemed to her. "I cannot tell you about
any events of the preceding day because there are none," the patient complained. "Don't you know how empty my days are,
don't you know that literally nothing happens? How can I tell
you what does not occur?" Finally, the psychiatrist pointed out
to the patient that her very symptomatology was the cause of the
alleged emptiness of her days. Then he asked the patient if she
took an hour or so to decide whether to put on the left or the
right stocking first; another hour to make up her mind whether to
wear the blue or the green dress; several hours to daydream about
the hatred and love she felt for the psychiatrist, members of her
family, or other significant people in her life. He inquired whether
she needed a further period of the day to daydream about her
longing for dependence, about methods of warding it off and for
disposing of the person or persons who instigated her sense of dependence. He then suggested that still more time had to be spent
in avoiding all kinds of taboos, such as touching allegedly con-
taminating material and in spying on those to whom she clung and
whom she hated. The patient admitted that this was so, and she
now understood that what to her had appeared as reluctance to
talk about her empty days was actually reluctance to report the
obsessional performances which filled these days. Subsequently,
she understood the crucial significance of the psychotherapeutic
investigation of the obsessional contents of her daily life. She also
recalled that some elements of her hatred against the psychiatrist
were the result of her anxiety connected with the exposure of her
obsessional preoccupations. Treatment then continued with the
discussion centering around the obsessional preoccupations which
filled the daily life of the patient. In due time this provided an
opening for the exposure of further obsessional personality trends,
subsequent to which she gradually dared to face further glimpses
of her anxiety, thus making the first step toward eventually resolving her obsessional symptomatology.

In using meaningful everyday material, the psychiatrist, of
course, must be careful not to allow his attention to dwell on this
to the point of overlooking significant historical data which patients may intentionally withhold. Patients may do so either be-

cause in their judgment this material is actually unimportant or because, wittingly or unwittingly, they wish to evade the communication of material which is more fraught with anxiety than are the daily occurrences.

It has been stated that indiscriminate use of free associations as a psychotherapeutic device is deemed to be of less significance, as a rule, than it was formerly. This in no sense means that the therapeutic use of associative thinking is barred from the psychotherapeutic scene. Its use is especially recommended in cases in which either patient, therapist, or both notice that they are at a loss in regard to the clarification of certain points under discussion or in regard to additional information needed for further understanding of unclarified difficulties, or if a patient's flow of thought runs dry and this situation cannot be remedied by direct questioning. An example in point will be given at the end of this chapter.

## 2. MARGINAL THOUGHTS, PHYSICAL SENSATIONS

Other tools mentioned as being helpful in such cases are to encourage patients to pay attention to and to verbalize marginal thoughts which may arise during a discussion of problems and general topics under scrutiny. The suggestion was also made that patients be trained to observe and describe physical sensations and symptoms as they arise and to notice both the present timing and the times and circumstances at which similar sensations or symptoms previously occurred.

The following report may serve as an illustration of the successful use of all three of these psychotherapeutic tools. A young woman patient complained of periodic attacks of hot flushes, accompanied by a sense of general paralysis and of feelings of numbness and nausea. While they lasted, her vision was blurred, objects and people looked distorted, large objects small, and vice versa. When such an attack occurred for the first time during an interview, the therapist inquired about the timing of its onset. The patient said that she was not able to time it or to identify in what connection it had occurred. She was then asked when and in what connection the initial spell of this kind had taken place. After some hesitation she recalled that it was while she was driving from her home to the college campus in a new Cadillac which her grandfather had just given her. She was sixteen at the time. After gaining this information, the psychiatrist, in order to break through her subsequent silence, suggested that the patient associate whatever came to her mind regarding the hot flushes themselves, their timing, and their connections. Following this suggestion, a wealth of material poured from her, all of it indicating her embarrassment about the lavish way her grandfather spent his fortune and because his extravagant expenditures on her set her apart and made her conspicuous in the eyes of her contemporaries and classmates. She was then asked to associate again to the timing and context of the spell that had occurred during the interview, and this time she was able to answer. The attack had begun while she was talking about visits she had paid to some people in rather reduced circumstances. During these visits she had discovered, much to her surprise, that these people were not at all unhappy because of their circumstances, despite the fact that her family had taught her that the contrary would be true. Again the patient was silent, and, since the psychiatrist felt that there was more on her mind, she was asked for further associations. None were forthcoming, so the therapist inquired about any marginal thoughts she might have had while giving her associations. After some hesitation, the patient replied that she most assuredly had had some thoughts on the side. They were to the effect that the psychiatrist was a bit plump without apparently being unhappy about it. This discovery was also contrary to what her mother had taught her because, according to mother, slenderness was supposed to be one of the roads to happiness.

Further associations to recurrent attacks of hot flushes during subsequent interviews with concomitant symptomatology made evident the fact that the hot flushes were an expression of the patient's discomfort about the wrong set of values given her by her grandfather and her parents, each in their own way. The recognition of their erroneous conceptions made her blush with embarrassment. Simultaneously, the realization of the extent to which recognition of her own environment had been blurred and her judgment distorted by her family's false teachings dawned on her with forceful dismay. Prior to treatment, the patient had not been aware of her feelings of disagreement with and opposition to her grandfather and her parents. She gave vent to them only through the channel of her physical symptomatology. The anxiety engendered by the expectation of the retaliative disapproval of the family had prevented her facing her rejection of their set of values. Through treatment she learned to develop sufficient self-respect to offset this anxiety.

Incidentally, the interpretive translation of her physical symptomatology, as above reported, was offered by the patient and not by the therapist. The psychiatrist would be very cautious about interpreting psychosomatic symptoms in terms of their appearance rather than of their etiology. For elaboration on this topic see pages 127–40. Needless to add, the possibility of an organic etiology of the patient's physical syndrome had been excluded by a thorough physical examination.

This example shows the resolution of a physical syndrome and of the originating anxiety by means of using the three therapeutic tools discussed in this chapter: directed associations, observation of marginal thoughts, and attention directed to the timing and context in which the symptomatology arose.

*3 keys to assoc —*

There are, of course, many more devices that can be used to elicit memories and other psychotherapeutically helpful data and to understand patients' communications (see also Augusta Slesinger, p. 57). Each psychiatrist must discover for himself which of these adjuncts are useful tools in his hands. The choice and usage of such devices depends, first, on the personalities of doctor and patient and, second, on the specific type of interrelatedness between them.

To give an example from my own experience: In eliciting emotionally significant childhood memories I have frequently found it most helpful to attempt to duplicate the interpersonal situation which I considered to have been responsible, in all likelihood, for the emotional experience in question. In these cases I may ask a patient not only for his own pet name but also for the first names or pet names of the significant people who seemingly participated in the situation. Of course, as many other psychiatrists do, I may also ask for a description of the room or place in which the experience took place. After that I call upon my own personal and professional previous experiences with similar situations with other people and patients in order to help me envision the one under scrutiny. Supported by this visual enactment, I then try to duplicate an alleged manifestation of a significant person's tone of voice, inflection, and vocabulary. For example, I may, mimetically, quote an oversolicitous mother and domineering wife saying to Robert, the father, in reference to Bill, their only son, who is my patient: "Hush, Bob honey, Bill knows that there is nothing more reliable than the love of his mother. So he will not even dream of doing thus and so if his mother tells him not to. He has inherited the fine brains of my father, so don't you try to advise him differently." See also Reich (128).

The patient's response to this reconstruction of a traumatic environmental childhood situation may be: "How did you know that?" Then previously repressed rage, resentment, grief, or anxiety, as the case may be, will come to his full recall, promoted by the doctor's reconstruction.

# CHAPTER VIII

## Interpretation and Its Application

INTERPRETATION has been mentioned variously in the previous discussion, and I shall now continue by elaborating upon its application. It has been previously stated that one may be or may become mentally stable to the extent of one's awareness of, or ability to become aware of, interpersonal experiences. If we assume this to be correct, then the basic psychotherapeutic necessity is to facilitate the accession to the awareness of previously dissociated and repressed material. This is done by interpretation.

By interpretation the psychiatrist translates into the language of awareness, thereby bringing into the open what the patient communicates to him without being conscious of its contents or of its dynamics, revealing connections with other experiences, or various implications pertaining to its historical or present emotional background. It is frequently not the actual events and happenings in the previous lives of patients to which they have become oblivious but rather the emotional reactions accompanying these events or engendered by them. Consequently, these connections and concomitant emotional experiences and not the events themselves often need interpretive clarification (6, 30, 37, 38, 40, 41, 46, 72, 84, 99).

This is shown to be all the more true, since one and the same event may have an entirely different emotional significance for any two people. These differing emotional reactions will depend upon the history and background of each person, the resulting total structure of their personalities, and their general patterns of life and living. Hence it follows that no interpretive psychotherapy is valid unless it is done with full and careful consideration of the interpersonal frame of reference specific to the personality of the respective patient. Bringing into awareness the contents of one or another single dissociation by report of pertinent data or by interpretive questions, as a rule, does not produce any curative effect.

When Freud made his initial discovery of the therapeutic effect of forcing recall of "forgotten" inner and outward events, it was his belief that a single interpretation might do the curative job. But he and his disciples had to revise this concept in order to have it fall in line with their subsequent therapeutic experiences. At the present time classical psychoanalysts as well as other psychoanalytically oriented psychiatrists know that the experiences which are brought into awareness by the psychotherapeutic endeavor will be repeated and will express themselves time and again in patients' various and sundry communications. The dissociated and repressed material which reveals itself to patients under treatment, in various connections—above all, in the realm of their relationship with the psychiatrist—must be tied together and worked through repeatedly, until awareness and understanding are finally transformed into constructive and curative insight into the basic patterns of a patient's interpersonal experiences (30, 38, 72, 99).*

In general, mental patients are unable to do adequate curative interpretive work without the assistance of, or at least indoctrination by, a psychiatrist. Should this not be self-evident to all readers, the following reminder is offered. My previous comments upon childhood amnesia also apply, *mutatis mutandis*, to adulthood: experiences which have been too painful or the recall of which would arouse too much anxiety have been dissociated or repressed in the course of patients' lives so that integration has not been possible. Repression or dissociation does not mean, however, the disappearance of this material but only the avoidance of its recall. That is the reason for its remaining unassimilated—lodged in the back of the patient's mind, as it were, like a foreign body. Most of the time it is impossible for patients to resolve these dissociations and subsequently integrate the previously "forgotten" material without the help of a psychiatrist. This is due to their fear of reliving the pain or of experiencing the anxiety which

* For good over-all information about the teachings of classical psychoanalysis and psychoanalytic psychotherapy see Ref. 79. For information about present developments in psychoanalytic theory and therapy see Refs. 5, 63, 64, 109.

accompanies the recall of dissociated and repressed happenings. Some people are capable of eventually resolving further dissociations by themselves, once they have learned how to do this under the guidance of a psychiatrist. Through his training and experience the therapist is equipped to do interpreting with and for the patient. He has learned to understand when and where, unknown to the patient, dissociated or repressed material finds means of expression, and when gaps in the patient's communications indicate that emotional material is being retained or withheld. A psychiatrist who is free of entanglements with his patients should also be alert to their inadvertent communications because he is not subjected to the fear of pain and anxiety which motivates the patients' dissociative and repressive processes.

In order to avoid misunderstanding, I would like to state at this point that, in speaking of the psychopathological effect of keeping emotional experiences from awareness, I do not mean to say that all dissociative or repressive processes are psychopathological in nature. The contrary is true. Man depends upon successful dissociations, repressions, and processes of "selective inattention" for the mastery of his psychobiological existence (147). It is the surplus of painful and anxiety-arousing emotional experience that creates psychopathological problems when barred from awareness (75, 76, 78, 117).

All schools of psychoanalytically oriented dynamic psychotherapy are in agreement that the processes of repression and dissociation from awareness of anxiety-arousing thoughts and feelings are one of the causes and signs of psychopathological developments. From this it follows that they all consider interpretive recall of repressed emotional material an integral part of intensive psychotherapy.*

There are great differences of opinion, however, among various

* For an over-all survey of the pertinent teachings of classical psychoanalysis and psychotherapy for psychiatrists and psychoanalysts see Refs. 16, 30, 31, 79, and 99. For an introduction to classical psychoanalytic thinking for the educated layman see Refs. 93 and 107. For information about some of the recent developments in psychoanalytic theory and therapy cf. Refs. 5, 6, 10, 63, 64, 84, 85, 102, 107, 108, 120, 147, and 152 for a helpful review of theory and therapy as viewed by the older non-Freudian psychoanalysts with literature references (109, 161).

schools of psychoanalytic thinking in regard to the genetic frame of reference in which interpretation is done and about the patients' selection of content matter for repression and dissociation. The genetic frame of reference of psychoanalysts is oriented upon Freud's basic teachings of the fundamental significance of the developmental history in infancy and childhood. However, there is a difference in the interpretation of the events and emotional experiences of the patient's early history, as determined by the psychosexual concepts of Freud versus the interpersonal interpretations of H. S. Sullivan (37, 55, 63, 64, 137, 147, 149, 151).* The patient's selection of subject matter for repression and dissociation, according to my thinking, is determined by the existing cultural standards governing his life. His medium of adherence to these standards is their acceptance by the significant people in his immediate environment and in his group.

To many people it is threatening to experience within awareness feelings, thoughts, and actions which are in contrast to these standards. These "forbidden" experiences may be unacceptable to the patient himself: they will be connected with the sense of expected disapproval by others, and so will arouse anxiety. Because of the anxiety-provoking character of culturally unacceptable experiences, the patient will attempt to bar them from awareness, to dissociate or repress them (54, 73, 147, 150).

At the turn of the century, when Freud discovered and began to teach the concept of repression, it appeared that sexual fantasies and experiences were the main entities and phenomena which had to be barred from awareness and to be resolved by interpretation. At the present time feelings of hostility, antagonism, and malevolence between any two individuals seem to be more subject to disapproval in our Western culture, therefore to more repression, than any other unacceptable brand of human experience and behavior. Could this perhaps be due to an attempt to counterbalance the generally accepted manifestations of hostility between the cultured peoples of our time, as manifested in the growing extent and cruelty of waging war?

In my experience, the psychiatrist will also frequently meet pa-

* Fairbairn's (26, 27) work marks an interesting transition from Freud's to Sullivan's concepts.

tients who are geared by the habits of this culture to keep friendly feelings toward people at large and toward the therapist from awareness and certainly from verbalization. This fear of realizing and expressing their own friendliness and therefore of accepting friendliness from others will frequently offer a clue to patients' interpersonal difficulties. I will discuss this topic at greater length in other connections.

Of course, there are various and sundry other unacceptable thoughts and feelings which may be subject to repression and dissociation in our culture and others. To mention only a few—the infantile overdependence of adults, interpersonal overpossessiveness or magic thinking, ideas of grandeur, etc. It seems sufficient, in this context, to mention these examples to illustrate the point that there is no universality regarding the contents of man's thought and feeling as they are subjected to repression and dissociation in various areas and cultures. It should be understood though, that I do not mean to infer that repression or dissociation of any of the groups of thoughts and feelings upon which I have exemplified separately, exclude concomitant repressive processes in any other realm of thought and feeling. This follows from the genetic or dynamic interrelatedness of most emotional experiences, and it is especially true for the frequent interrelatedness of sex and hostility. Before offering any interpretation, a psychiatrist should listen to his patients without harboring preconceived ideas about the genetics or the contents of their pathogenic dissociations and repressions. This will greatly facilitate the correctness and therapeutic validity of his interpretations.

Unfortunately, some therapists may attempt interpretive psychotherapy with the preconceived idea that there are universally valid rules governing alike, for all their patients, the genetics and the selection of contents for dissociation and repression. Under the pressure of the expectations of the psychiatrist and because of the eagerness of their dependent and suffering patients to comply and to please, patients may frequently produce what their psychiatrists are looking for. However, that is no proof of the correctness of these interpretations; but it evidences the innate competence of human nature. It is due to this competence that some mental patients are capable of using the helpful dynamisms inherent in all psychotherapeutic exchange for the benefit of their striving toward recovery. It may be said that this sometimes does happen regardless of the validity of the interpretation.

## 1. WHAT TO INTERPRET

### a) CONTENTS OR DYNAMICS

In the preceding chapters comments have been offered to the effect that interpretive attention should be focused mainly upon the revealing vicissitudes of the patients' interpersonal operations with the psychiatrist and more specifically upon the manifestations of their negative transference and upon their security operations. I will further elaborate on these topics in the following two sections.

As a rule, part of the resistive and security maneuvers of patients should be brought into focus first (see pp. 107–18). Special attention must be paid to the investigation and interpretation of the genetic experiences and dynamic processes underlying the patients' manifestations. This is because these processes as well as the contents of the manifestations themselves may be outside patients' awareness (see pp. 74–111). As has been said, the general trend in the development of psychoanalytic psychotherapy at the present time is toward replacing the first type of interpretation with the second one. Subsequent to effective genetic and dynamic interpretation, understanding of the therapeutically relevant hidden meaning of the contents very often takes care of itself. This has been illustrated by the example given in Part I (p. 19). However, there are no fixed rules and regulations about the question of when to emphasize genetics and dynamics or when to pay attention to content interpretation. The choice of the interpretive approach in each instance and with every patient must be determined by the nature of the psychopathology of the patient, that is, his specific means ("dynamisms," "mechanisms") of trying to dispose of past and present anxiety-producing emotional experience.

Originally, interpretive psychotherapy was developed for use with neurotics only (31, 37). The special modifications for its application to other types of mental disorders is still in the process of being developed (65). One way of clarifying various psychopathological entities is to look at the diversities in the defense mechanisms used against the rise of anxiety into awareness. This determines the distinctive psychotherapeutic approach to various disorders. To put it in very broad terms and only for the purpose of outlining the differences of therapeutic approach that are known at the present time, the following can be said. The psychoneurotic's response to experiences connected with unbearable emotional pain and anxiety is to bar from awareness the experience and the events which promoted it. Therefore, when he tries to talk to the psychiatrist about pathogenic experiences, he is liable to use the means of expression characteristic of dissociated and repressed experiences without knowing it. When doing this, he will not understand the actual meaning of his communications unless the therapist translates, that is, interprets their meaning for him.

It should be stated in this connection, though, that the general spread of knowledge of what Freud has called the "language of the unconscious" has increased the alertness of the average educated neurotic to the covert implications of his manifestations. Freud predicted this development when he first taught psychiatrists and their patients to become aware of and to understand the hidden meaning of these manifestations. This fact is among the causes which have helped to decrease the psychotherapeutic need for content interpretation and to develop the present therapeutic trend of concentrating more upon the interpretation of dynamics (130).

With the schizophrenic, interpretation of dynamics and genetics is *the* approach needed. One of the schizophrenic's responses to excess emotional pain, anxiety, and distrust of others is to withdraw his interest from the outside world and to live in a private inner world of his own, i.e., on a level of thought and feeling which is different from that of the psychiatrist who listens to him. Hence he expresses himself more often than not in a private language of his own or in a way which sounds like mere tenuous allusions to the nonschizophrenic listener. However, the schizophrenic patient himself, as a rule, is aware of the content meaning of what he communicates about his inner experience in this private world, no matter how cryptic his communications may sound to the listener. The listening psychiatrist may need an interpretation of the meaning of the manifestations of his schizophrenic patient, but it is a rare occurrence for the patient to need help in understanding the immediate content meaning. The patient, though, does have a prevailing need for help in becoming aware of and in learning to understand the genetic and dynamic background and the unknown implications of his conflicts and his symptomatology (114, 160). If the psychiatrist understands the private language of a schizophrenic patient, he must evidence this by adequate responses. As previously stated, it is, however, redundant, as a rule, "to point out" to the schizophrenic patient the content meaning of his communication, which to him is no secret within the framework of his own schizophrenic modes of thinking and expression. By this statement I do not mean to advocate, however, that the therapist exclude reformulations of the contents of vague and indirect or symbolic schizophrenic communications and insights. They frequently become therapeutically meaningful to the patient only when he hears them clearly and directly reformulated in the rational language of the therapist. The question of what to do if the psychiatrist does *not* understand the meaning of the schizophrenic communications has been discussed in Part I (pp. 17–19) (68).

Patients who try to cope with their anxiety in terms of manic-depressive mood swings need active interpretive help in all three of the areas—contents, genetics, and dynamics—and, above all, in regard to the significance of their operations with the psychiatrist. Moreover, it is mandatory for the psychiatrist to take into consideration that patients suffering from manic-depressive mood swings move very slowly in the psychotherapeutic process. This slow tempo is due to the very tenuous nature of their interpersonal relationships; their lack of ability for correct observations, registration, and report of interpersonal experiences; their lack of interest, early training, and talent for introspective observation and understanding; and their misleading inclination for play acting (71, 92).

In psychotherapeutic work with psychopathic personalities, it is indicated that great thriftiness be used with interpretations in all areas. These people make an attempt to counteract their insecurity, that is, their anxiety and their self-contempt, by compulsively paying lip service to the acceptance of interpretations offered. They try their hand at doing some seemingly astute interpreting of their own as an intellectual maneuver designed to placate the psychiatrist. They are driven to do this by their defiant need to please. Their intellectual alertness and their marked sensitivity to the expectations of others equip them for it far too well for their own good. It is a far cry from this pseudo-understanding to actual therapeutically valid insight. However, this does not indicate agreement with the current view of those psychiatrists who believe that the road to insight and cure is not accessible to these people. But the psychiatrist must safeguard against interfering with these patients' gaining real insight by offering them too many interpretations without realizing the specific difficulties in their making constructive use of them. Care and discrimination regarding timing and number of interpretations is more of the essence with psychopaths than with any other type of mental patient. Perhaps these examples will suffice to illustrate my point that the choice of interpretive approach must be co-determined by evaluating the type of mental disorder specific to the patient under treatment.

There are no unfailing, generally applicable rules that can be offered, notwithstanding the generally valid regulations governing interpretive work that have been and will continue to be outlined in this book. In the last analysis the question of how to go about the process of interpretation depends to a great extent upon the psychiatrist's and the patient's personalities and upon the general nuances of their psychotherapeutic collaboration. All nonprofessional, social intercourse between two people of any given culture is governed by the rules and regulations generally accepted in their culture. Yet the interpersonal exchange between any two people engaged in the same type of social exchange is bound to be difficult, no matter how rigidly both couples follow the accepted set of social regulations. This difference is determined by the specificity of the personalities of the two people concerned. The same is true for the professional exchange between the two participants of the psychotherapeutic process—the mental patient and the psychiatrist.

I will therefore try to illustrate the two possibilities of interpretation of contents and dynamics by giving some examples of both. At the present phase of psychoanalytic experience, I feel that this is all that can be done in an attempt to convey the principles and the interpersonal atmosphere of this part of the psychotherapeutic process. The first example has been selected as an illustration of the need for genetic interpretation in the psychotherapeutic procedure with a schizophrenic.

A patient suffered from severe jealousy and envy of the younger sister of the family, who was six years her junior. She entered the psychiatrist's office one day, looked into the mirror, shook her head as though in disgust, and said, "My sister Lizzie is in nurses' training now." Lizzie was endowed with the conventionally accepted charm and attractiveness of the very pretty American girl as we know her today. These attributes were very pleasing to the patient's mother, a metropolitan society woman. The patient herself was a well-built, strikingly attractive, intelligent-looking young girl whose type of good looks, however, did not appeal to her conventionally minded mother. Until the birth of the very pretty infant sister, the patient had been the only girl in the family. She had been the pet sibling of five older brothers and the favorite child of her parents. The arrival of the baby sister deprived her of the role of the family favorite which she had occupied for the first six years of her life. It was especially mother, the most significant figure in the family group, who, from this time on, shifted her affection and interest from the patient to the newcomer. As the sister grew up, she promised to become the great social asset of the family, who would thereby glorify her mother. Being dethroned this way at the age of six was among the pathogenic factors determining the later rise of the patient's mental illness.

The patient's looking into the mirror discontentedly and her comment upon Lizzie's being in training for a useful occupation versus her spending her time in a mental hospital were an expression of this early traumatic experience. It was as if she were saying, "I envy Lizzie because she is pretty and I am not, and because she is usefully occupied and I am not."

The psychiatrist who would feel called upon to interpret this manifestation might consider telling the patient, in so many words, about the above-mentioned meaning of her combined gestural and verbal communication. This would be an error. As has been pointed out, it may be taken for granted that a schizophrenic patient is fully aware of the factual contents of his communication; that is, this patient would know that the meaning she had conveyed to the psychiatrist was, "My sister is prettier and more useful than I am." She might not realize the implication of the pathogenic envy and jealousy aroused in her from early childhood by her sister's alleged superiority. Interpretation, therefore, if offered at all, should deal only with the latter aspect of the patient's communication.

The question of whether or not this interpretation should be offered will be dependent upon the timing of the patient's communication in relation to the place it holds in the total psychotherapeutic process and in the doctor-patient relationship. Should the time not be ripe for the genetic interpretation, the reaction of the psychiatrist, for the time being, would be to evidence his understanding of the factual meaning of the patient's communication by an adequate response. He might say, for instance, "There may be many people who would not prefer Lizzie's type of good looks to yours." This remark, however, should by no means be made by a psychiatrist who had not seen the sister. Otherwise the patient could only take it as a sign of meaningless reassurance, which could be detrimental to her therapeutic relationship with the doctor. If the therapist's statement is backed up by personal knowledge, it serves the double purpose of proving to the patient that the psychiatrist has grasped her meaning as well as creating a frame of reference for use in later interpretation. Another type of useful answer might be, "What are your future plans for training or occupation when you leave this hospital?" Either response will serve the purpose of demonstrating to the patient that the psychiatrist has heard her expression of concern about the alleged unfavorable outcome of a comparison between herself and her sister.

For many months following this incident, the patient gave repeated evidence of her envy and jealousy of her sister. She was not capable of realizing it, however, because the anxiety aroused in her premorbid childhood days was too great. This anxiety had been fostered by the realization of "forbidden" feelings, such as envy of one's younger sister. In the social milieu of the patient's family group such feelings were totally unacceptable.

Eventually, the patient's wish for change and recovery had grown sufficiently that she was ready to face her envy and jealousy. Her interest in curative insight and her ability to accept her own moral evaluations, quite independent of those of her family, were concomitant with this wish for change. Despite this trend toward health, the patient's life-pattern of being envious and jealous of other women repeated itself strongly in the relationship with her female therapist. Therefore, it was too difficult for the patient to admit her insight to the psychiatrist, much less to accept interpretive comments about it from her. Hence it would have been premature for the doctor to comment on it at the time of the above incident. Discussion of her envy had to be postponed until the patient was finally able to accept it. This happened in the following way:

During one of the psychotherapeutic interviews she discovered a newly acquired *Encyclopaedia Britannica* in the psychiatrist's office. The patient asked the doctor to select a topic about which the patient could read to her. This was done, and then the patient was asked to select a topic herself. She chose an article on Memling, the Dutch painter. The psychiatrist was convinced that the patient's choice was not accidental, but she had no clue to what determined it. Feeling her way, she asked the patient if she had ever seen any of the original Memlings. The patient's eager response brought forth the following story. The patient, her parents, one brother, and her sister Lizzie had been to see the original Memlings at the art museum in Bruges. As they were ready to leave, her brother went to see about their triptyques, leaving the car parked on what appeared to be an unused railroad track. Without warning, a train approached, and the family waiting in the car became panic-stricken. It was the patient, then only seventeen, who had the presence of mind to jump into the driver's seat, turn on the ignition, and get the car off the track just in time. The parents, suddenly relieved of their panic, hugged and kissed Lizzie. Her story ended here.

The patient did not deem it necessary to mention that her parents, in their joy and relief at the rescue of their younger daughter, failed even to express their gratitude to the older one, who had saved their lives. This would have been the time for the psychiatrist to have pointed out to the patient the envy and jealousy engendered in her by her parents' behavior. Her reluctance to admit it prior to this event because of her envious competition with the psychiatrist could also have been pointed out then. This was not necessary, however, because the patient herself gave evidence of being fully capable of realizing her previously dissociated feelings. In fact, she seemed to offer her story as a means of admitting her agreement with the psychiatrist's repeated related statements. Therefore, the therapist simply repeated the last words of the patient's report, "And then my parents hugged and kissed Lizzie." This was sufficient in itself to convey to the patient—again, by an adequate response rather than by verbalized interpretation—that the doctor had "heard" her finally accept the fact of her envy and jealousy. From then on, the patient's and the doctor's psychotherapeutic collaboration could include their mutual dynamic knowledge of the patient's envy and jealousy of her sister. She could also see the parataxic repetition of such feelings toward the therapist and others and the fact that the realization of these "forbidden" feelings was one of the roots of her anxiety.

Incidentally, I wish to mention—even though it has no direct pertinence to the topic under discussion—that the patient's disgust at the sight of her mirrored image also meant that she was disgusted with her looks, irrespective of the judgment of the family and of the unfavorable comparison with her sister. Like many other patients who are a prey of their emotional difficulties and of their unacceptable feelings, the patient thought she was "ugly" because, in her judgment, she was inwardly ugly, as it were. If for no other reasons, she considered herself so because of her envy and jealousy of Lizzie, dim as the awareness of these feelings had been at the time of this first event.

The next two examples are illustrative of the need for content interpretation of the reports of two neurotics. Both were unaware of the meaning of the contents of communications which furnished an important clue to the understanding of the nature of their problems. These examples are also selected in order to illustrate a specific way in which the psychiatrist can gain understanding of the content meaning of patients' communications, should he fail to do so merely by the process of listening. The first patient gave an account of the following repetitional experience. Upon various occasions he felt called upon to take a deep breath, fill his chest to capacity, and retain the air as long as possible. Concomitant with this, he felt that something connected with his body should be eliminated. The whole experience was described as extremely pleasurable. It was reported at the time of his wife's third pregnancy.

The psychiatrist sensed from the puzzled, intrigued, and gleeful tone of voice in which the report was given that it might be quite important if its meaning could be understood right then and there. Having no idea what it meant, it occurred to the doctor to apply a device for gaining a clue, the use of which may be recommended in order to gain insight into the language of the body. The doctor tried to duplicate the patient's physical experience. She took a deep breath, filled her chest to capacity, and retained the air as long as she could. As she tried to dispose of something connected with her body, she felt at a loss. She then decided that the patient must be talking about disposing of some part of his anatomy which she could not sense in connection with hers. Hence she assumed that he was referring to his penis. After that, she understood what it meant to the patient to fill one of the cavities of his body to capacity, to enjoy the feel of it, and to be gleefully puzzled and intrigued. The patient tried to experience himself as a pregnant female. This interpretation proved to be correct. The patient accepted it avidly, as one would accept a great revelation, and commented instantly upon his envy of his wife, whose privilege it was to experience a third pregnancy. This birth-envy was subsequently discovered to be an important factor in the psychopathology of the patient.

Aside from the technique of interpretation or from the specific problem of the patient under discussion, I would, in this connection, like to draw attention to the danger of the psychiatrist's understanding the problems of his patients exclusively in the light of his culture. In this patriarchal culture we are inclined to think of man's superiority to woman and women's envy of it. Women's envy of men, which Freud understood as biologically rooted in their penis-envy and whose cultural determinants were subsequently understood, has a strong correspondence in men's birth-envy. An exemplification of this is offered by this patient's experience (14, 37, 53, 55, 75, 83, 103, 115, 159). Psychiatrists must be able to detach themselves from the prejudices of this civilization so that they may be able to discover and to familiarize some male patients with the existence of their envy of women or of their birth-envy and its possible psychopathological concomitants (see also pp. 32–38 and sec. 3, pp. 202–5).

From conversations with colleagues and students, I infer that there is general unfamiliarity with the device of purposeful imitation of a patient's physical experience in order to gain understanding of their cryptic communications about it. Therefore, I would like to give a second example of a treatment history where this device proved to be helpful to me. A patient gleefully related that his favorite position was to sit with his legs twisted about each other. The emphasis put on this narrative made me feel that there must be more to it than met the eye. I tried sitting down and twisting my own legs, and I discovered that I could not do so. I found, however, that, in the course of attempting it, a sense of self-involvement would have conveyed itself to me had it not been counteracted by my concentration upon the patient's problems. Prompted by this feeling, I ventured to ask the patient about the degree of his interest in himself and others of his own sex. It evolved that the patient was an overt homosexual and that he had tried so far to keep this knowledge from the psychiatrist.

Incidentally, this experience is an illustration of the previously mentioned concept that man's tendency toward health is ever present. Adverse conscious trends in his personality, however, interfere at times with its effectiveness. The patient had consciously tried to keep the fact of his being homosexual from his psychiatrist. Yet he felt motivated to tell the conclusive story of his favorite position, thus giving the therapist an opportunity to uncover the symptom. To be sure, something in the patient must have dimly realized what he was doing. His motivation toward health was stronger than his wish to withhold important information from the psychiatrist. I trust the reader will understand the therapeutic legitimacy of this attempt to grasp the manifestations of a patient by directive imitation versus the nondirective identification which has been previously denounced in a different context (Part I, pp. 7–8).

The following report of a schizophrenic patient offers a case in point for the previous recommendation of the therapeutic usefulness of reformulation of a patient's own insights by the doctor.

This patient told the psychiatrist that he had been the only boy and the idol not only of the immediate family but also of the entire family group. This continued for the first four years of his life, when he was irretrievably dethroned by the arrival of a baby brother. Suddenly and for reasons beyond his grasp, the attention and affection that had been given him in such overabundance was transferred to another child. He felt helpless and desperate. Finally, one day, so the patient reported, he took his baby brother out of the crib and carried him to the open window of a fourth-floor apartment, with the intention of throwing the baby out of the window. At the last minute he could not bring himself to do it. Upon hearing the baby cry, the mother came into the nursery to see what the trouble was and to comfort the baby. She recognized that the baby's distress was of the older brother's doing and proceeded to scold him. Apparently, it had not occurred to her that there might have been distressing reasons for the older boy's disturbing the baby.

While telling the psychiatrist about this incident, the patient was well aware of the fact that the worst part of the experience had been the mother's lack of insight into the state of agony which he had suffered because of the temptation to kill his brother. His only comment, however, about this part of the experience was a vague statement about his mother not having evidenced any understanding of his part in the situation. Reformulation of the experience by the therapist was indicated here, regardless of whether this was an actual experience or a childhood fantasy. Central attention had to be focused upon the worst part of the patient's experience by rewording his report and by stating plainly that his mother had utterly failed him at a time when the little boy had needed her most.*

Another example of helpful reformulation stems from the experience of one of our associates with a severely disturbed schizo-

* Perhaps most readers will realize that the nonverbal interpretive response versus worded interpretation of the psychotics' communications constitute a recommendation which is different from the new attempts at doing psychotherapy with schizophrenics about which John Rosen has recently reported. He responds to a schizophrenic's communications with immediate, solid interpretations (along the line of the libido theory and of the psychosexual concept of the patient's developmental history; cf. p. 180). From Rosen's reports it appears that his method has made him very successful in bringing his patients out of the state of acute psychotic disturbance very quickly—as a matter of

phrenic girl. This patient reported to the psychiatrist with whom she had been working over a long period of time: "I moved up and down and up and down in my bed and was quite upset. I don't know why you told me that I had to wear spikes while doing this!" This patient had been recently moved from the most disturbed ward of the hospital to a less disturbed one. On this occasion she had made the resolution to stop manual masturbation. She was as mixed up about her own sex as most schizophrenics are. The psychiatrist, to whom the patient had previously given information about both these facts, reformulated the patient's statement for her as follows: "So there was sexual excitement and relief from jumping up and down in your bed. And you were not sure whether or not one had to be a boy ["spikes"] in order to jump around that way. And you *do* feel that you need the psychiatrist 'to tell you about it.' "

Many of the examples offered as an attempt to clarify the question of interpretation of contents or dynamics have been taken from the experience with psychoanalytic psychotherapy with schizophrenics. This seems legitimate to this writer because much of what psychiatrists originally learned in their therapeutic dealings with these patients is now also considered applicable to neurotics (149). There is another justification for this procedure in addition to the reasons which have been mentioned in the Introduction. What little we know to date about intensive psychotherapy of psychoses stems from the experience with these introspectively gifted people. At present they also constitute the greatest percentage of hospitalized and ambulatory mental patients.*

---

fact, markedly more quickly than it occurs, as a 'rule, when using the interpretive suggestions I have offered. However, there is not as yet enough data to show whether or not the method of shocking the patient out of his disturbed psychotic state, as it were, may create difficulties in the total course of the illness which may interfere with the later course of treatment.

Part of Rosen's unquestionable success in speeding the emergence of the patient from his acute psychotic symptomatology seems to be due to his temporarily entering the patient's delusional world with participant action and that he then gives interpretations while in the role of the patient's delusional partner (135, 136).

* This viewpoint is in contrast to the concepts of Melanie Klein. Her British psychoanalytical school takes its basic lead from Klein's interpretation of her experiences with manic-depressive patients (92).

*b*) Transference and Parataxic Distortions

Continuing the discussion of what to interpret, I shall now give further consideration to the vicissitudes in patients' relationships with the psychiatrist, first, to the transference phenomena. "Transference" in the most general sense of the word means transferring to and repeating early patterns of interpersonal relatedness with present-day partners as they take place in everyone and therefore also in every patient. Hence we try to understand part of a person's psychology and of a patient's psychopathology by investigating the history of his early formative experiences in interpersonal relationships. This way we gain the necessary information and knowledge about the significant partners in his early formative years (see also the discussion of history-taking in "The Initial Interview," pp. 45–69).

Transference in its special application to the therapeutic process naturally means transferring onto the therapist, as a present-day partner, early experiences in interpersonal relatedness. Such significant carry-overs from people's early relationships with the parents of their childhood, of course, will also affect their later relationships with their family doctor, dentist, minister, etc. Even the mere anticipation of consulting any kind of qualified helper, including the future psychiatrist, may pave the way for the development of transference reactions (133). The following reasons make the investigation of interpersonal relationships with the psychiatrist especially important for therapeutic purposes. First, the psychiatrist is an active observer of and a therapeutic participant in the patient's psychotherapeutic experience, but he does not share the experience as such. Therefore, the psychiatrist is free to conduct the interpretive investigation of patients' transferred interpersonal experiences with him *in statu nascendi*, as an observer who does not become involved. Second, the patients' early formative experiences and present interpersonal patterns as transferred onto the therapist can be seen and investigated as if under a magnifying glass. This is because of the great transitory interpersonal significance of the therapist for patients. Third, special significance must be attributed to those experiences which are repeated with the psychiatrist without a patient's being able to realize their repetitional character or to recall the original underlying experiences.

Of course, the reason for the special relevance of interpretive scrutiny of these forgotten experiences is the same as the one previously given for the general therapeutic relevance of bringing dissociated and repressed material to awareness. Dissociated early experiences are barred from participation in the growth and maturation of the rest of the personality. Their evaluation and interpretation in the minds of patients are therefore essentially uninfluenced by the increased ability for judgment and evaluation which people acquire after these early, now dissociated, experiences have occurred (see also "The Initial Interview," chap. v, about dissociated and repressed memories). Patients are neither aware of this fact nor cognizant of its causes. As a result, present-day persons and interpersonal situations will be misjudged, incorrectly evaluated, and parataxically distorted along the lines of the patients' unrevised, early, dissociated experiences. This will be evidenced with specific clarity and emphasis in patients' relationships with the psychiatrist.

These distortions of people and relationships are responsible, of course, for part of patients' emotional difficulties in living. The central part of all intensive psychotherapy is therefore the interpretive clarification of the connection between a patient's early patterns of interpersonal relationships and his present experiences. Dissolution of parataxic misjudgments can best be done through the medium of investigating the distortions in patients' interpersonal experiences with the psychiatrist. In this context I would like to offer a formulation of H. S. Sullivan. As soon as a patient has understood *one* parataxic distortion and accepted it as such, there is a glimmer of hope for a successful outcome of the psychotherapeutic process (147).

Freud has emphasized the special therapeutic significance of these problems by his statement that the term "psychoanalysis" may be applied to every type of psychotherapy which recognizes the problems of transference and resistance, the basic importance of the "Unconscious" and of the early developmental history (51). However, the previously mentioned modification of the frame of reference in which interpretation of transference phenomena is understood by many psychiatrists now (pp. 4–6) also calls for modifications of the method of their interpretation.

Great emphasis has been placed by classical psychoanalysts upon patients' recognizing and resolving their Oedipal attachments to the parents of their childhood through re-experiencing with the doctor their transferred sexual feelings of love and hatred. However, if the Oedipus complex is not considered universal and if the unresolved Oedipus constellation is not a ubiquitous etiological factor in the pathology of mental disorders, then it follows that there is no reason always to find transferred Oedipal love and hatred for the psychiatrist in the interpretive picture (cf. chap. viii, pp. 80–84). This statement does not imply that the psychiatrist may not find many developmental histories of neurotic and psychotic patients who love the parent of the same sex and hate the other. But, in line with the previously mentioned revision of the psychosexual concept of the developmental history, we find this love by no means to be always sexual in nature. Consequently, this hatred is seldom of the nature of sexual rivalry (see pp. 6 and 83). In my experience the wish for closeness and tenderness with the beloved parent and the envious resentment about the authoritative power of the hated one, both without recognizable sexual roots, constitute a more frequent finding in childhood histories of healthy, neurotic, and psychotic people than do their sexual Oedipal entanglements with the parents of their childhood (14, 60, 109).

Frequently the reports of patients about their early attachments to their parents may lend themselves to sexual misinterpretation. However, in evaluating these data, the psychiatrist should keep in mind the possibility of patients' difficulty in expressing feelings of friendliness toward the doctor and his own problem of accepting them. People of this Western culture do not seem to find it too difficult to talk about sexual attachments, falling in love, etc., but, as previously mentioned, many of us are reluctant, if not afraid, to speak about the friendly, tender, asexually loving aspects of our interpersonal relationships (Part I and pp. 83–84). This holds true not only for adult relationships but also for feelings of attachment to the parents of one's childhood as viewed and reported by adult patients. Moreover, the psychiatrist's own fear of a friendly give-and-take, if not recognized, may encourage these misconceptions.

Furthermore, the educated and psychoanalytically well-read patient of this era who comes to see a psychiatrist will try to comply with the alleged concept that the doctor will expect to hear about his Oedipus complex. Misrepresentation of patients about the early relationships with their parents and misinterpretation by the doctor of the data offered may result from both these sources. The possible tendency of the psychiatrist to discuss the Oedipus complex rather than to scutinize the tie-up between the patient and himself was discussed in "The Psychiatrist" (Part I).

The psychiatrist who follows these deductions will naturally pay close attention to the vicissitudes of the patients' relationship with him, including the experience of love and hatred from real or alleged Oedipal sources. But he will not intentionally push or force patients into re-experiencing these feelings with him, as was frequently done in the early days of psychoanalysis (155).

Interpretive emphasis regarding transference experiences is now placed mainly on the investigation of the patterning influences of the transferred early experiences and on the concomitant parataxic distortions, less so on the experiences of love and hatred for the therapist per se. As these previously dissociated experiences are repeated with the therapist, they are brought to awareness and utilized to help patients with the process of reality testing on the experiential level of their present chronological age (31, 38, 39, 40, 72, 99, 133, 141, 156).

Not all "transference" reactions have to be pointed out in so many words. This becomes necessary only if they are accompanied by marked and repetitional distortions which threaten to becloud or slow down a patient's ability to recognize and appraise interpersonal issues in reality. However, it is always of paramount significance that the psychiatrist be alert to their recognition whenever they occur. This task is more complex than it may appear upon first sight. The previously mentioned reluctance of a psychiatrist to recognize and discuss details of patients' interpersonal relatedness to him does not constitute the only possible cause for a doctor's possible failure in accomplishing it. There is also an objective fact which holds the threat of interference. It is only rarely that a patient manifests only "transference" or only "real" feelings toward the psychiatrist. They are intermingled most of the time.

This fact is among the causes for the complexity of the doctor's task in disentangling and in correctly recognizing all of a patient's transference reactions. Yet it is of great therapeutic significance that the psychiatrist succeed in doing so. This suggestion holds for all manifestations in the doctor-patient relationship which show marked repetitional characteristics. In addition to love and hate reactions, immature attitudes of transferred overdependence must be brought clearly into focus, irrespective of their immediate or postponed therapeutic utilization.

As outlined before, the realization of patients' transference feelings must, at times, serve as a guide in conducting the psychotherapeutic procedure. If psychiatrists are alert to this necessity and follow this suggestion consistently, transferred love reactions to therapists will be resolved automatically most of the time in the course of the total psychotherapeutic process. Their dissolution will no longer constitute the great psychotherapeutic task so frequently mentioned in the early psychoanalytic literature (31).

In the psychoanalytic literature of more recent years it is recommended with increasing frequency that the therapist refrain from commenting on patients' loving relationships with the doctor and that he pay more interpretive attention to its hating aspects (128). I am inclined to indorse this suggestion wholeheartedly. It is especially advisable to keep it in mind with regard to schizoid and schizophrenic people, with their fear of and longing for close relationships. They will not be benefited by the doctor's commenting upon the positive manifestations of their relationship with him. Sometimes, however, they may get help, as other patients do, if the hateful or malevolent aspects of their relationship with the doctor are pointed out to them.

Generally speaking, though, the same holds true for the therapeutic handling of either pole of the relationship. If the therapist is comfortable as recipient of both sides of patients' relatedness to him, the interpretation of experiences resulting from and concomitant with their reactions of hostility may turn out to be as redundant as that of their loving relatedness to him. As a rule, patients themselves will speak about their hatred in its real and in its transference aspects, as it becomes therapeutically indicated, if and when they work with a doctor whom they sense to be undisturbed by their transitory hatred (cf. Part I, pp. 22–24).

Active interpretation of patients' hostility will be necessary, though, if and when it is part of their attempted security operations with the doctor. Freud's recommendation that priority be given to the interpretation of resistance over that of the rest of a patient's manifestations should be repeated in this connection (Part I and pp. 107–18). Sullivan's recommendation of giving interpretive priority to patients' security operations should be mentioned here in the same vein (p. 188). The extensive discussion of resistance and security operations will be taken up in the next section.

Some illustrations follow which are designed to clarify the understanding of the remarks on the development of the concepts and of the psychotherapeutic use of transference reactions and parataxic distortions.

A patient opened the psychotherapeutic session one day by commenting upon the lovely spring day, the sunshine, and the birds' singing. The therapist interrupted this small talk by suggesting that she talk about therapeutically more important material, upon which the patient burst forth in anger, saying, "First you doctors suggest that we become more spontaneous and direct in our exchange with you and then if we follow your suggestion you try to cut us off." The therapist immediately realized that this previously extremely withdrawn and inarticulate patient was right, he admitted that she was, and he apologized.

Six months later, upon entering the psychiatrist's office for her psychotherapeutic interview, this patient looked at a flower vase and commented, "What a lovely vase. Look at the sun's colorful reflection in it." Fortunately, the doctor recalled the first incident. With this in mind, he assumed that the patient was testing his reaction to her remark about the colorful reflections of the sun in his vase. She wanted to find out whether or not he had actually meant what he said, when he had previously apologized after cutting short her talk about the weather and the sunny day. This could be brought into the open, and it became one step in the patient's understanding that not all people would let her down by their lack of reliability as her parents had; that is, her reality testing through an experience with the doctor helped her to do away with a significant parataxic misevaluation of other people.

When the discovery of transference phenomena was first made, though, psychoanalysts understood that this type of remark should certainly be interpreted as an expression of a patient's positive transference. "She likes or loves the doctor and expresses herself in terms of admiration for his vase," was then the psychoanalyst's interpretive conclusion.

Regardless of whether or not in any given case the implication of this type of remark by a patient is true, psychiatrists are now more interested in investigating whether such remarks may have more important therapeutic implications. This indeed proved to be true in this instance.

The second example illustrates the operation of a parataxic distortion in a patient's dealing with her therapist because of her unresolved tie-up with her mother. This patient told the psychiatrist in one of their interviews that she was planning to go to a party that night. The doctor, pleased with the progress indicated by the patient's decision, responded by saying, "Fine." At the next interview the doctor heard that the patient did not go to the party. Asked about the reason, her reply was that the doctor had said, "Fine," exactly the way her mother had been prone to do. Frequently, when the mother did not want the patient to do this, that, or the other, she did not dare to interfere openly. Therefore, the patient had also distrusted the motive behind the doctor's "Fine." After verbalizing this, she understood the parataxic character of her reaction. The patient's giving up the party in response to her interpretation of the doctor's motive is an illustration of a special type of transference, "acting out." A general discussion of the therapeutic approach to acting-out processes follows on pages 120–27.

The third example is that of a patient who visualized his blue-eyed female psychoanalyst as bearded and brown-eyed. That is, his distorted picture of the psychiatrist coincided with the appearance of his dead father, who had been brown-eyed and had had whiskers. Concomitantly with the distortion of the psychiatrist's looks, he, of course, also misinterpreted the doctor's reactions and behavior as being similar to childhood experiences with his father. Many of these childhood experiences had never been revised and revaluated, because they had been dissociated up to the time the patient had entered the therapeutic relationship with his doctor. The interpretive clarification of this transference experience at last made a revision possible. Subsequently, this revision became part of a general revaluation of the patient's interpersonal reality.

So far, I have given examples to show the importance of transference processes and parataxic distortions determined by tie-ups between patients' childhood experiences and those with the therapist. Previously, I made the point that, wherever possible, psychotherapeutic considerations should also include the interpretive investigation of the patients' transference experiences in terms of their presenting problems and their recent crises situations. The following example illustrates how that can be done. A woman patient in her late thirties came to see the psychiatrist. She had just terminated the fourth in a succession of unhappy love affairs. Her attitude toward the therapist was characterized by a marked degree of deference, hero-worship, and overacceptance of, if not submissiveness in the presence of, his authority. This attitude alternated with an equally marked display of a great sense of superiority.

Very early in life this woman had developed a great sensitivity to the marital problems of her parents. She had learned to protect and to take sides with father against mother and vice versa. That is, she had assumed, as it were, the parental role of both. Of course, at the same time there was an intensive longing simply to play the role of a young child, denied her because of her parents' marital difficulties. So she was torn between her longing to be a child, acceptant of authority and capable of admiring the adults, and her actual role of being a superior parental figure in the family group.

Both attitudes repeated themselves in the two facets of her relationships with her lovers. Unable to establish relationships on a basis of mutual equality, she knew only how to play the superior parental figure upon whose protection her parents had called or that of the submissive child who was ready to admire authority in the role for which she longed and which had been denied her in her childhood. As a result, she consistently became entangled with people whose personalities, background, or age group were such that they elicited the patient's living out one of these two alternatives, yet blocked her from establishing a mature, mutual relationship on her present age level. Because of this she had also modeled her relationship with the psychiatrist along the same psychopathological prototype. Subsequently, her interpersonal difficulties in her childhood and in her previous and in her recent crisis situations could be brought to her awareness through the medium of this transference experience. Her insight into this process became a significant starting point for the therapeutic dissolution of this pattern.

The last exemplification of the therapeutic significance of transference reactions stems from a patient who was deprived of her mother's exclusive love and her father's concentrated attention by the birth of her younger sister. The only adult who was available for the establishment of a mutual relationship at that time was a governess. Therefore, the patient developed a markedly possessive, clinging relationship to this woman. This patient asked the psychiatrist for an explanation of the following apparently contradictory behavior which she had observed in herself that day on the way to his office for the interview. "As a rule," she said, "I don't seem to want to come to see you. Then, when I do come, I don't want to be reminded of the fact that you also see other patients. I want to be able to think that you belong only to me." The interpretive investigation for which the patient had asked showed that the reason for her not wanting to come to see the psychiatrist was that her special nurse would spend time with others for the duration of the patient's interview with the doctor. Hence the reason for her not wanting to come was the same as her wish to be able to think that she was the psychiatrist's only patient. In both situations the lonely adult patient was repeating the pattern of clinging possessiveness which the lonely child had first learned to develop in her relationship with her governess.

When the patient first heard the interpretation for which she asked, she became rather upset and responded by saying, "How dare you tell me such a terrible thing?" Then she quieted down, commented that she knew the doctor was right, and stretched out on the couch. Then she remarked upon how comfortable she felt with the psychiatrist, who had opened her eyes to this problem in her interpersonal relationships. After that she said, "I know very well that my seeing this does not mean it is gone, but at least I understand it, and that is the first step." The fact that the interpretation for which the patient had asked contained, by implication, an evaluational attitude toward her behavior on the part of the psychiatrist may have decidedly contributed to the intenseness of her emotional reaction. This assumption seems all the more justified, since patients are, of course, generally inclined to use the psychiatrist as the representative of their own extrapolated conscience, hence as their moral guide. Incidentally, this is one of the traps set for the pleased and flattered psychiatrist to develop a countertransference to the patient which may becloud therapeutic issues (see Part I). The legitimacy of the patient's statement that her intellectual understanding of the situation would not do away with it once and for all will be proved in the discussion of "The Process of 'Working Through'" (p. 141).

Before concluding these remarks on the interpretive therapeutic use of the doctor-patient relationship in its real and parataxic aspects, a note should be added on its final outcome when treatment is terminated. Any person who has been useful to another in the process of solving emotional difficulties in living may become and remain invested with a legitimate amount of importance in the mind of the person who has been relieved of his lonely suffering. This holds true regardless of whether the help is given by a friend or in a professional situation. Such evaluation need not be parataxic. It may be useful and constructive, as is every legitimate evaluation and every adequate emotional response of a patient. Therefore, I do not agree with the classical psychoanalytic viewpoint expressed by Lou Andreas Salome's statement that the therapeutic resolution of a mental patient's transferred and real overattachment to the physician must result in the former patient forgetting his previous doctor and his relationship with him (7). I believe the doctor's fear of mutual friendliness, upon which I commented at the beginning of this chapter, is responsible for this unrealistic conception.

Feelings of resentment against a psychiatrist who has not been able to be useful can be equally realistic, especially if the psychotherapeutic process was maintained too long after efforts had proved to be futile. Again, psychiatrists' fear and insecurity in the presence of a patient's legitimate criticism and resentment may be at the root of the doctor's attempt to deny the legitimacy of the antagonism of these frustrated patients. Labeling it "parataxic" or feeling that it may be the outcome of patients' resistance or negative transference is a powerful defense in the hands of a frightened psychiatrist.

The patients' state of overdependence upon the psychiatrist which has been discussed here and on pages 35, 84, and 190 will be dissolved concomitantly with the process of growth and maturation which is psychotherapy, unless the therapist enjoys and cultivates the dependence of his patients for his own needs. Verbalization, clarification, and acceptance of these realistic aspects of the doctor-patient relationship should most assuredly be part of the psychotherapeutic process. They must not be neglected in favor of the interpretive clarification of its parataxic aspects. This topic has been previously mentioned in Part I (p. 36) and will be taken up again in chapter x, pp. 188–94.

### *c*) SECURITY OPERATIONS, RESISTANCE

It has been repeatedly pointed out that one central difficulty of most mental patients is constituted by their feelings of anxiety and insecurity; by their need for acceptance and prestige; and by the defenses they use in pursuit of evading the first and obtaining the latter. Scrutiny of the defenses which patients use in their relationship with the therapist and with others is therefore an integral part of psychoanalytic psychotherapy. Patients use various types of defenses such as isolating techniques, procedures of "undoing," etc., in accordance with their specific psychopathology (54). As previously mentioned, the symptoms themselves are an expression of their anxiety and of their defenses against it. I will elaborate upon this topic later. The special defenses of which people avail themselves in nontherapeutic interpersonal situations are also used by mental patients in their dealings with the psychiatrist. To mention only a few of them: sudden shifts in the stream of thought or change in the tone of voice, rate of speech, body tension, or motor activity; fatigue; embarrassment; the need to be plausible, perfect, or apologetic. In the case of the psychotherapeutic situation, attention should be paid to the repetitional, the "transference," character of patients' defensive manifestations. Subsequently, their retarding function in treatment and their paralyzing and isolating influence on the patients' interpersonal relationships with the doctor and with others should be brought to their attention and eventually to their recognition.

Because of these reasons, I have repeatedly commented in previous chapters upon the significance of the investigation of the patients' security operations, their ego-defenses against the psychiatrist and the psychotherapeutic process. The significance of the therapeutic procedure was first pointed out by Freud in his writings on psychoanalytic technique (37, 38, 40) and in "The Problem of Anxiety" (54). In line with the growing psychoanalytic understanding of Ego-psychology and of Sullivan's operational conceptions (102, 147, 151), it has found increasing acceptance in recent years by classical psychoanalysts and by other psychoanalytically oriented psychiatrists (79a).

The following example may illustrate a complex type of defense used by a patient in her dealings with the psychiatrist and its therapeutic utilization. A patient broke through prolonged periods of compulsive silence by asking the psychiatrist questions about his personal life. The therapist did not fall into the trap of interpreting this as an expression of the patient's curiosity engendered by her attachment to him. He understood that the same anxiety which had kept the patient silent so far was now operating in her verbalizations. Therefore, his response to the patient's questions about him was to the effect that, should she remain interested, he would have no objection to answering these questions at some later date. For the time being, however, he was more interested in and therefore wished to instigate the patient's interest in the reasons prompting her to replace therapeutic curiosity about herself with concern about the doctor's personal affairs. After that the psychiatrist could demonstrate to her that the anxiety she felt in her dealings with him, which she tried to ward off at all costs, was the reason for her remaining silent or talking about him instead of discussing her problems. Subsequently, this became a starting point for the therapeutic investigation of the same pattern used in the patient's interpersonal dealings with people at large. This patient had been reared to lead the life of a self-sacrificing, kind, generous, and charitable person. As a result, she had developed intense feelings of resentment and hostility, primarily against those who had forced upon her the yoke of this self-sacrificing attitude. After that her "kindness" became a reaction formation to the resentment and the destructive fantasies against those close to her and quite frequently against the recipients of her charitable generosity. This was her "secret," of which she was only dimly aware, however. Fear of her own disapproval as well as of the disdain of others prompted her to hide the "secret" as best she could. Therefore, the patient had assumed the obsessional pattern of evading an answer to any personal question asked her, whether it was by a friend or a mere casual acquaintance. Her automatic response to any personal question was to ask in return a personal question which expressed her concern with the affairs of the friend or acquaintance.

The interpretation and understanding of her use of the same type of security operation with the therapist, as she emerged from her long silence, constituted the first step toward the patient's resolving her obsessional pattern of being "good" and her compulsive need to hide that she was not. She eventually learned to accept the fact that she was not called upon to be more kind and generous than her fellow-men. Following this insight, her hostile and destructive fantasies, as well as the compulsive need of hiding them behind her obsessional self-denial, also subsided. It was from repeated thorough scrutiny of recurring security operations with the therapist, similar to the first one, that the patient ultimately learned to develop a wholesome pattern of mutual give-and-take with others. This undermined her destructive fantasies, the anxiety subsided, and ultimately the patient became free enough to let go of her obsessional security operation of hiding behind the screen of an artificial overconcern for others.

One other type of security operation which plays a great role in the patients' dealings with psychotherapy and psychiatrists is the dynamic process known as "resistance." "Resistance" means the reactivation, outside of patients' awareness, of the motivating powers which were responsible for the mental patient's original pathogenic dissociative and repressive processes. This resistance manifests itself in the course of the psychotherapeutic process as reluctance against relevant communication and against the acceptance of interpretive

resistance

clarifications or its possible concomitant therapeutic changes. The same source which motivated the patient's original dissociative and repressive processes, that is, his anxiety, is also the main reason for this resistance. In other words, the patient is resistive to psychotherapeutic collaboration and interpretation for fear that the anxiety which the material in question originally barred from awareness may be reactivated by the interpretive dissolution of the dissociations and repressions.

Resistance is as much a process outside the patient's awareness as the original dissociating processes are. It is up to the psychiatrist to be constantly alert to its recognition as it arises. The interpretation of processes of resistance should constantly be included in the psychiatrist's and the patient's collaborative efforts at interpretive clarification whenever the pertinent presuppositions are fulfilled, which will be discussed later.

Further possible causes for patients' resistive interference with free productions, collaboration with, and acceptance of interpretive clarification are the following: first, a patient may be afraid to follow the psychiatrist's suggestions because, if he does, it may presuppose and express closeness to and acceptance of the therapist. As previously mentioned, this seems dangerous to many people in this culture in general and to many patients, especially schizoid and schizophrenic people, in particular. As we have repeatedly seen, these patients are always afraid of the rebuke which may follow such acceptance and of the reactions of hatred which rebuke on the part of the other person will engender in them.

Another group of patients is reluctant to collaborate and actually to accept beneficial interpretive clarifications for fear of becoming obligated to the psychiatrist by accepting anything beneficial from him. They are the patients who may have been raised by parents one or both of whom have presented a bill of demands and obligations in return for every favor they did for their child.

To illustrate: A catatonic patient who had been mute over a long period of time responded one day to the psychiatrist's attempts to interest her in resuming verbalized communication by a sudden outburst, saying, "I don't know why you continue trying, don't you see that I am not interested?" The therapist replied by saying that he was aware of the patient's lack of genuine interest but that he felt justified in trying to get the patient interested in spite of herself or to help her operate for the time being on the therapist's belief that it might be worth the patient's while to try to recover. Seeing an expression of incredulity and impatience on the patient's face, the therapist continued by saying that he had no personal stake in the question of the patient's recovery other than the legitimate interest of fulfilling the professional obligations and responsibilities incurred when accepting the job of doing psychotherapy with the patient. Furthermore, he added, he would not consider it a waste of time and energy to have tried to interest the patient in resuming a creative life on the outside, even if his efforts were destined to fail because the patient's interest could not be aroused. At this point the patient was seen to relax markedly and to be able to hear the therapist, who continued by emphasizing that the patient, in her turn, incurred no obligation toward the therapist because of his efforts to be useful to her.

The next day the patient took up communicative exchange with the psychiatrist. Much later she confirmed the psychiatrist's assumption that she could do so because he had assured her that no debt would be incurred by her if she accepted his endeavors on her behalf and that this attitude was in contrast to all her previous experiences with the significant people in her environment, especially the parents of her childhood. This exemplification of one of the causes instrumental in arousing a patient's resistance in her work with the doctor illustrates, at the same time, the previously mentioned function of reality testing inherent in the doctor-patient relationship.

There are other ways in which patients' anxiety-born reluctance to collaborate with the attempt of the therapist at interpretive clarification may be evidenced, some of them outside of, others within, awareness. The patient may develop a defensive "selective inattention" to the suggestions or interpretations which the psychiatrist has to offer, or he may "draw a blank" and feel that his ability to listen or his capacity to concentrate is completely wiped out. Again, a patient may try to depreciate the interpretive questions of the psychiatrist by making light of, or poking fun at, the psychiatrist or the psychotherapeutic procedure or himself as the subject of the procedure. Others may try a facetious approach, which the sophisticated patient may handle with such skill that the therapist may easily be led into a discussion of the contents of this type of response instead of recognizing and commenting upon the patient's resistance as the motivating power behind his facetiousness. Less sophisticated patients may try to evade the interpretive approach to their own problems by talking about the psychiatrist instead of submitting their problems to interpretive psychotherapy or instead of listening to interpretive suggestions.

In the psychoneurotic, such talk should immediately be discouraged as irrelevant, and its significance as resistance should be brought to the patient's awareness. Attention should be paid to content matter, such as alleged interest in the doctor's personal life, only if its very choice permits specific clues regarding the patient's psychopathology. The previously reported case of the patient who repeated an old pattern of silence about herself and verbalized concern about others in her security operations with the therapist illustrates this (see pp. 108–9).

The same holds true for the attempts of psychoneurotic patients to delay interpretive psychotherapy by discussing at great length their relationship with the doctor, especially its positive aspects. These patients may also try to impress upon the psychiatrist the fact that they cannot talk frankly with him for fear of losing his love and appreciation. In the terminology of classical psychoanalysis, their positive transference is used in the service of their resistance. Wherever the patient's comments on his relationship with the doctor are clearly a resistive maneuver, they should be discouraged by the doctor. This may be done by expressing doubt of their therapeutic validity or by a display of boredom rather than by an attempt to interpret what the patient knows. Interpretation of this type of transference productions, which are clearly motivated by resistive tendencies, may more frequently than not amount to a mutual oral flirtation under interpretive disguise.

In the case of more seriously disturbed patients, however, talking about the doctor is frequently the only way these people can overcome their initial reluctance to speak at all. Such patients may not talk about the psychiatrist in particular, and they do not try to convey the idea that things concerning him are important to them. But they may do it as a means of the inevitable evasion to which some of these very aloof and remote patients must resort, as they first break through their muteness. At other times, they may well express something pertaining to their own problems by allusion, imagery, or figurative speech, as they seemingly talk about problems pertaining to their doctor's life. The psychiatrist will have to depend upon his empathic sensitivity to discern when such talk about him is motivated by resistance and should therefore be stopped and interpreted, and when it constitutes the cautious attempt to resume interpersonal communication. If the latter is the case, the therapist must try to use the patient's remarks about him as an avenue by which to slowly approach the patient's own problems. It would not be wise to jump to conclusions about the doctor-patient relationship at the time of the first emergence of an inarticulate patient from a long period of silence, and it would be equally wrong to discourage him from verbalizing this material. Either attitude would be liable to throw the patient back into silence.

One formerly mute patient, for instance, resumed verbalized contact with the doctor by commenting upon having heard that the psychiatrist was giving lectures downtown. The psychiatrist responded by saying that his lectures were quite pertinent to the patient's own problems, as he was lecturing on the topic of the assets which were frequently found concomitant with, or even as an outcome of, the liabilities of people suffering from mental disorders. There followed a vivid exchange on the topic itself and on its relevancy for this musically talented patient. As they conversed, the psychiatrist consistently related things to the patient's problems. Beginning with this incident, interpretive psychotherapy could be carried on without further interruption by episodes of muteness, until her ultimate recovery was accomplished several years later.

Another misleading type of resistance is expressed in what appears to be some patients' hopelessness or insurmountable grief about their worthlessness or about the unconquerable degree of mental disorder, so that psychotherapeutic endeavor is unwarranted or sure to fail. Further devices which patients may use in the service of resistance, without their being aware of it, might include the following means: resistive silence, alleged inability to recall the topics of interpretive clarification from a previous interview, missing scheduled interviews with obviously lame excuses, attempts at evasiveness, flight into the production of irrelevancies or the use of what are supposed to be "free associations" to lure patient and therapist away from what really occupies patients' thinking. This last group of resistive measures may be spotted and recognized by the psychiatrist more easily than the preceding ones.

Long-drawn-out discussions of the question of whether or not the therapist is the right person for the patient to work with, in respect to personality, age, sex, experience, brilliancy, astuteness, patience, etc., are another device frequently used by patients to delay interpretive clarification of anxiety-arousing material. The same holds true for many other types of futile argumentation and for all attempts to drag the psychiatrist into argumentative exchange.

Somatic symptomatology may also be used to draw the attention of the psychiatrist and of the patient himself away from an unwelcome topic of discussion. As a rule, the *type* of symptomatology will be expressive of, or a response to, the evaded topic of discussion. The rise of psychosomatic symptomatology has therefore to be considered interpretively in its double significance, as an expression of the conflict-arousing issue and as a means of evading its clarification within awareness (see also pp. 133–34).

There is another form of resistance with which some readers may be familiar from their own experience in psychoanalytic treatment and training. Sometimes patients readily profess to the intellectual acceptance of an interpretive suggestion which seems to make great sense. Then they hedge and subsequently try to nullify such acceptance by the statement that they can see the justification of the interpretive suggestion intellectually but they cannot follow it up emotionally. There are three possible reasons for this kind of statement. One: the therapist has created in the patient's mind a hazy, romantic conception of the expected emotional response to a meaningful interpretation. The patient then may debunk a valid experience and acceptance of an interpretation by comparing it unfavorably with the hazy, extravagant connotation of what he allegedly ought to feel in connection with understanding the interpretation. Two: the patient may hold onto the belief in an alleged lack of emotional reaction to the new interpretive clarification, as a means of barring it from anxiety-provoking acceptance and integration. Three: there is the possibility of the actual dissociation of the emotional reaction as a means of resisting creative insight, the reason again being the anxiety connected with the acceptance of the interpretive clarification per se and with the fear of changes in their interpersonal operations, which the patients' insight may presently promote or necessitate in the future.

In addition to the general resistive measures and security operations mentioned thus far, all specific dynamisms which are used in various types of mental disorders to maintain dissociations and to ward off anxiety may be repeated as resistance and as security operations.

Obsessional patients, e.g., may make use of their repetitive, argumentative, manipulative, and compulsive ways of interpersonal behavior. They may also use the promotion of never ending doubts about trivia, their pedantic rigidity, and the surliness and malevolence which is theirs, as a means of counteracting the therapist's attempts at using an interpretive approach designed to make these patients face their anxieties.

The schizophrenic may use his powers and skills for aloofness and withdrawal into a hallucinatory world, his regressive dynamisms and negativistic attitudes to ward off the attempts of the psychotherapist to approach his anxieties interpretively.

Transfer of blame, fantasies of being persecuted by the psychiatrist, and withdrawal into a private world of secret grandeur will be used by the paranoid person to block an effective interpretive approach to his anxieties.

Psychoneurotics may use the following dynamisms and symptoms as their specific means of nonacceptance of therapeutic collaboration: "selective inattention," alleged inability to accept interpretations, distortions of the communications of the psychiatrist, escape into overemotional responses and dramatizations, development of conversion symptoms.

A special comment on handling obsessional types of defenses may be added here because the problem of breaking them down is most complex and difficult. The character of the interpersonal operations of the obsessional as power actions is frequently skilfully disguised. Many of them are of a distinctly autistic, proto-

taxic, magic nature (11, 147). These magic power actions are designed to disguise the exceedingly deep-rooted insecurity of these
people. Since it constitutes the main defense in their struggle for
psychological survival, the attempt to break it down entails the
threat of arousing great anxiety. If the psychiatrist keeps in mind
what the dynamic significance of the resistance of these people is,
he should be able to resist the tendency to be taken in by their attempts at getting him entangled into arguments and other types of
mutual power struggles (cf. p. 121).

Another afore-mentioned resistive mechanism which presents
the psychiatrist with a difficult problem in interpretive psychotherapy is patients' negativism. Unlike other types of resistance,
negativism, as a rule, cannot be helpfully approached by interpretation. Needless to say, attempts at forcing its breakdown by rational argumentation will not work either. The only therapeutically useful reaction to negativistic blocking of psychotherapeutic
collaboration should be statements of the psychiatrist in the vein of
"That is, then, as far as we can get today; I hope you can talk about
this (or answer the question) (or give me your reaction to this
interpretation) in the near future." Following this, the negativistic
patient will sooner or later take up the topic in question, sometimes
immediately, at times several days or weeks later, at other times
many months hence.

In order to understand this, we have to remember one of the
possible causes of negativistic behavior. Negativism is an attempt to
get attention, used by people whose insecurity hinders them in
relating themselves significantly to their fellow-men in more
pleasantly effective ways. H. S. Sullivan illustrates the dynamics
of negativism in terms of the negativistic behavior of a little child
who is sent to bed. If he goes silently, no one will give him any
further thought that evening, much less speak to him. If he stamps
his foot, shouts, and refuses to go, he will immediately become the
center of attention. Negativism in mentally disturbed adults is a
regression to, or a duplication of, this behavior. Therefore, interpretation and argumentation will not break it down. Avoidance of
forcing the issue by expressing one's willingness to wait quietly, as
described above, is the only means of doing away with the point in
fact which calls out negativistic attitudes (147).

To illustrate: a patient requested, time and again, that she be dismissed from the hospital, while psychotherapy was progressing successfully. On the basis of various data which the patient had previously offered, the psychiatrist assumed that the patient's urge to leave the hospital might be determined by some experience related to her father. Therefore, one day he responded to the patient's question as to what he wanted her to talk about, with the suggestion that she give further information about her father and her relationship to him. "What am I supposed to do now?" was the patient's indignant response, "operate like a slot machine? You say 'talk about father,' and I am now to go ahead and talk about father." The psychiatrist's answer was that he realized that the patient would not be able to comply with his request immediately.

Many months later, when the patient was appreciative of an extra interview which the therapist gave her to meet a special need of the patient, she showed the therapist a photo of her late father and made the comment that he died in a mental hospital. She left it up to the therapist to guess the implication of this information. The patient's repeated, urgent requests for dismissal from the hospital, although in her own eyes and those of the therapist psychotherapeutic progress was satisfactory, were due to her fear that she, too, might die in the mental hospital, unless she left it previous to such impending doom. Obviously, the patient knew this was the reason for her fear of prolonging her hospital stay, when the therapist initially asked the interpretive question about the patient's father many months earlier. At that time the therapist's hope of getting conclusive data along these lines was met with negativistic blocking. This could be overcome only much later, by the therapist's not asking for it and at a time when he had given the patient a special sign of attention by seeing her spontaneously for a non-scheduled, special interview.

To conclude the section on psychotherapeutic dealings with resistance and security operations of the patient, a few remarks may be added on the timing of the interpretation of these phenomena. Security operations and resistive maneuvers will be produced time and again for the duration of the treatment situation. By and large, they should currently be pointed out to the patient as soon as a workable doctor-patient relationship has been sufficiently established to assure that the doctor's suggestions may be heard by the patient and be meaningful to him. Also the relationship with the therapist must be sufficiently established so as to preclude the patient's mistaking the doctor's interpretations of his resistance for a reprimand. The patient must be prepared to understand that the interpretation of his resistance does not carry with it the connotation that he is responsible for its appearance, as though it were a case of intentional blocking within his awareness. This is not said with the thought in mind that there are not patients who occasionally show signs of intentional stoppage of therapeutic collaboration with interpretive procedures. However, these reactions of advertent blocking are not referred to as "resistance."

There is one further important consideration which the psychiatrist should bear in mind when making decisions about the proper timing for his interpretations of security operations. A state of sufficient general integration should be reached by the patient to enable him, without breaking down, to carry the amount of anxiety which may be temporarily aroused as the interpretation of his security operations leaves him without his previous defenses against the anxiety which is mobilized by the therapeutic process. This is in line with the statement made in the chapter on the "Initial Interview" that there is no therapeutic merit in the doctor's being instrumental in a mental patient's temporary breakdown. Further suggestions about the correct timing of these interpretations may be deduced from the general discussion of the timing of other interpretations in section 3, pp. 150–53.*

### d) INTENTIONAL BLOCKING

Not all the patients' interference with psychotherapeutic collaboration is due to resistance, that is, due to a type of reluctance which is outside awareness. There are also, of course, episodes of intentional blocking in practically every patient who undertakes intensive psychotherapy. This conscious reluctance to collaborate psychotherapeutically may be wittingly expressed by practically all the devices of which patients make use for their security operations and for the resistive processes which are outside their aware-

* For literature about resistance see all references given about the technique of psychoanalysis (31, 35, 36, 37, 38, 39, 72, 79a, 99, 128).

ness. Lack of communication, lack of interest in following the suggestions of the psychiatrist, "drawing blanks" which interfere with any give-and-take in psychotherapeutic exchange, and failure to appear in time or at all for scheduled psychotherapeutic interviews are the most common means of intentionally defeating the psychotherapeutic process.

The following is an enumeration of some possible causes for such purposive blocking. These causes may be due to a patient's reluctance to admit that he is suffering from mental symptoms or to his reluctance to admit personality trends, difficulties in the family, or character trends of family members of which he is ashamed. Again, intentional blocking may be engendered by patients' reluctance to accept the authority of an expert or by their fear of changes within themselves and in their overt interpersonal relationships, as they may be produced by psychotherapy. Another reason for patients' blocking communication may be created by their lack of experience, hence lack of belief in the possibility of verbalized communication with another person (the doctor) on the level of human equality. Also, patients may distrust the motives of the psychiatrist; or their hostility against people in general—therefore also against the psychiatrist—may be greater than their wish to get help. Again, their lack of self-assurance, which is so frequently coupled with the wish to defeat others, along with them the psychiatrist, may be greater than their alleged hope for useful therapeutic collaboration. Finally, their reluctance to spend the time and the money required for intensive psychotherapy may be stronger than their wish to obtain help.

The psychiatrist should first try to help such patients to overcome what—within their awareness—interferes with their therapeutic collaboration. He may convey his sympathetic understanding and try to encourage verbalization. If, however, the patients' blocking during the interview or their failure to keep appointments, etc., do not yield to such endeavor after some time, the psychiatrist is then justified in the assumption that the pressure which these patients suffer from their mental symptoms is not great enough to cause them to relinquish their prejudices against the psychiatrist and the psychotherapeutic procedure. This being the case, such patients should not be discouraged from discontinuing treatment, at least for the time being. They are welcome to return for treatment, and they will do so when there is sufficient pressure, and therefore a strong enough desire for treatment and relief, to induce them to overcome their reluctance against abiding by the rules which govern the psychotherapeutic procedure.

### e) "Acting Out"

One more among the psychotherapeutically important phenomena which may be used by patients in the pursuit of transference reactions as well as of resistance and other security operations are processes of "acting out" instead of verbalizing interpersonal experiences. More specifically, "acting-out processes" are the actions and activities in which patients engage—during the psychotherapeutic interview and outside it—as an expression of, or a reflection upon, their relations with and their attitude toward the therapist and the psychotherapeutic process and, through this medium, as an expression of their interpersonal problems at large. The investigation and interpretation of these reflected actions and activities inside and outside the therapeutic interview have to be kept in the focus of interpretive attention for the entire duration of the psychotherapeutic process.

In addition to these "acting-out" processes in the strict sense of the word, the activities and the behavior of most patients who are under psychoanalytic treatment also show some general reflections of their interpersonal experiences in the treatment situation. Although most of the time the latter are too vague, diffuse, or tenuous to make their therapeutic use rewarding, it is always worth while to have them in mind while listening to and evaluating the patients' presentation of data of their current life. The patients' presentation of intercurrent events and the events themselves if co-determined by the patients' attitudes may be inadvertently influenced by the way in which they experience and evaluate the personality of their doctor and the mutual aspects of the doctor-patient relationship.

Acting out, of course, is not encouraged by the psychiatrist, who is mainly interested in the investigation of verbalized material. But it happens, irrespective of all the discouragement which it may be given. The observations, investigations, and interpretations of the patients' acting-out processes can frequently be used as a means of resolving his resistance and its retarding consequences. They may also be used as a contribution toward discovering and making the patient gain understanding of his interpersonal problems, as in the following example.

A lonely woman patient became engaged to an unsuitable partner each time that the psychiatrist, the only person with whom she had meaningful interpersonal contact, took a vacation. Previous to her acting out her loneliness in this way, the patient had not been able to accept as a problem the fact of her being lonely, nor could her interest be sufficiently aroused that she would enter into a scrutiny of the cause of her aloneness and her loneliness. The whole experience was too much under censorship because of the attitude of this culture toward it. A girl is not supposed to be or to feel lonely or alone. She is supposed to be popular. If one is lonely, one is a failure. It is one's own fault.

The patient finally faced her loneliness after a third meaningless engagement during the vacation of the psychiatrist. The realization of the symptomatological meaning of the acting-out engagements as devices to counteract her loneliness was, of course, of the greatest therapeutic significance. Only after the patient had achieved the recognition of the symptomatological significance of her acting out could she become interested in entering into the interpretive clarification of its genetic reasons and of its dynamics, which then could eventually produce curative effect.

Such action, betraying a patient's symptomatology in its relatedness to the psychiatrist and to the psychotherapeutic process outside the therapeutic interview is not so frequent as patients' acting out during the interview. Time and again in an interview, patients try to express themselves in terms of actions rather than in verbalized communications, as in the following case of an alcoholic patient.

This patient had been given a medical order confining him to the hospital grounds until some of the emotional problems which drove him to compulsive drinking had been better recognized and worked through. This patient was one of those unhappy people who have been brought up to live in an icy interpersonal environment, in which the significant adults feel that useful interpersonal exchange can be only in terms of manipulative power actions. Because of this manipulative atmosphere at home, the patient did not know of any other interpersonal approach. Therefore, he repeatedly evaded any attempt to abide by the doctor's administrative decisions. For a long time he fought every one of them, tooth and nail, by word and by action. The compulsive need to act out by manipulating the psychiatrist appeared to be greater than his tendency toward health. After having gone through some greatly frustrating binges with severe social and legal implications, the patient allegedly realized at last that it would be wise for him to be confined to the hospital grounds. Only a few days later he found himself compulsively ready to re-enact his old pattern by succeeding in manipulating the psychiatrist into restoring his privileges. The rationalization was that he badly needed to go to the dentist. The suggestion of the therapist that this might be a face-saving excuse was refuted with a display of severe suffering from painful sinusitis and tooth-ache.

As the dentist confirmed the psychiatrist's suggestion by his negative findings, the patient became extremely upset and emotionally shaken. At that moment the therapeutic insight dawned on him that he was acting out with the psychiatrist his lifelong pattern of fighting and manipulating others and of keeping the upper hand in the fight. The nonexisting sinusitis and dental trouble, which he had used in pursuit of his attempt at acting out his need to use his powers to convince the therapist, finally brought to his awareness what he had been resistive to seeing, in spite of all the preceding verbalized therapeutic endeavor.

Needless to say, one such insight did not change his tendency to deal with the therapist in terms of power manipulations, and a real break could be inaugurated only after the occurrence of several similarly enlightening experiences. But the fact remains that the patient first caught onto his deep-rooted manipulative interpersonal integration, by being faced with it in the course of acting it out.

Other examples of acting out during the psychotherapeutic process may be shown by patients who get angry. Instead of verbalizing their anger, they may feel called upon to throw things at the psychiatrist, etc. A further example in point is an exhibitionistic patient who may begin to undress or to exhibit his genitalia during the therapeutic interview or a patient who actually or allegedly falls in love with the therapist. He then wants to talk love, if not to make love, instead of investigating this interpersonal experience in the making, in its quality as a transference experience and in its relatedness to his past experiences and to the present pattern of his interpersonal relationships. These people are also among the patients to whom psychiatrists refer when they speak of patients who put their positive transference in the service of their resistance (cf. "Security Operations, Resistance," p. 107). An additional way of acting out frequently used by neurotic patients is to cling to actual or allegedly bodily complaints as a rationalization for requesting a physical examination time and again, without its actually being warranted by their somatic condition.

The therapeutic usefulness of acting-out processes during the interview must be evaluated in terms of the type of patient concerned. In neurotic patients they have to be considered, as a rule, as an expression of resistance against interpretive clarification, since what is acted out lends itself, by and large, much less easily to interpretive investigation than what is verbalized. In spite of the examples quoted to show the possibility of making successful interpretive use of acting-out processes as they inevitably occur at times, the psychiatrist should immediately try to discourage all acting-out processes in the neurotic.

Ferenczi, one of the most impressive leaders in the early years of psychoanalysis, followed a different course. He was convinced, as are all psychoanalysts, that the clarification of early infantile and childhood experiences are of paramount significance to patients. He invited patients to re-enact their experiences with him, believing that these transferred reactivations would speed therapeutic understanding and dissolution of the traumatic validity of these experiences (31, 72, 99, 155, 157, 158). My objection to this suggestion stems predominantly from the danger implicit for many psychiatrists of losing track of their role as participant observer by becoming a gratified participant co-actor in relation to the patient's infantile needs. I feel more strongly opposed to it from this standpoint than from anything else that has been said for verbalization versus action. This objection is similar to those discussed later regarding sexual experiences with patients.

In rare selected cases, the acting-out of neurotic patients may be encouraged as a therapeutic or as a diagnostic device, as in the following situation: an artist of high repute who had discontinued sculpturing after the birth of her eagerly expected first child came to see the psychiatrist for a state of depression. She felt paralyzed in all of her activities and skeptical about her creative abilities both as a mother and as an artist. She thought that abandoning her artistic career was what she owed the baby, yet she resented the prospect of doing so. Moreover, those of her friends who were young mothers themselves reminded her of her duties toward the baby, while her artist friends impressed her with her obligation to art.

The psychiatrist was cognizant of the patient's depression and paralysis, but felt that the problem as outlined by the patient did not ring true. Therefore, this patient was invited to "act out" her alleged problem through effigies, as it were. It was suggested that she bring photos of her baby and reproductions of her sculpture to a psychotherapeutic interview. The expectation was that a display of and comments upon the two conflicting aspects of the patient's life, might help to clarify the issues, as indeed it did. While showing and explaining her photos and reproductions, the patient discovered, with the doctor's help, the real nature of her problem. She could see that it was not constituted by the alternative between being a good artist or a happy mother but by the alternative between being an artist or a dissatisfied wife. Marital conflicts were at the root of her depression and paralysis. Subsequently, both she and her husband entered psychoanalytic treatment.

The therapeutic attitude toward acting out in psychotics must, of necessity, be different from that toward the acting-out processes of neurotics. The mute psychotic may frequently act out what he cannot express in words. At times actions are all that is available for psychotherapeutic work with these inarticulate people. It can be discouraged only gradually in psychotic patients, therefore, as their inarticulateness subsides.*

As the psychiatrist tries to discourage the angry neurotic's acting out, the patient may attempt to maintain his acting-out attitude as resistance by accusing his therapist of being afraid of him, or the

---

* Cf. in this connection my experience with a mute catatonic reported in Ref. 66.

exhibitionistic patient may defend his position by accusing his therapist of undue prudishness. The psychiatrist should never be misled by such maneuvers for the maintenance of the patient's resistance. He should not respond to such "accusations" by defending himself or by discussing whether or not he is cowardly or prudish, as the case may be. Instead, he should convey to the patient that the discussion of the doctor's fear or prudishness is beside the point, since he and the doctor are concerned with the patient's, and not with the therapist's, analysis. This attitude is especially recommended for the psychiatrist's dealings with those neurotic patients who use acting-out processes in an attempt to jeopardize the professional character of the doctor-patient relationship. These patients may try to get a rise out of the therapist, as they challenge him by the display of markedly hostile or sexually seductive behavior. "If I can't make you love me, I want you at least to get mad at me," was the way one patient explained this mechanism. "If you get mad, I know at least that you care somehow. I just have to break through your professional detachment and indifference."

In response to such behavior the therapist should avoid the temptation of seeing and depicting himself as a paragon of equanimity. Assuming any such role is a challenge to the patient, who may set out to demonstrate that this role is not foolproof—and he may or may not succeed in doing so. The doctor will be more helpful by stating that the patient may well be able to make him angry or irritated by being nasty or making a nuisance of himself per se and, more so, by delaying the progress of psychotherapy. The patient may then be encouraged to think over whether or not all this is worth his while.

The psychiatrist may evidence to these patients his lack of interest in and his boredom with their attempt to wreck the psychotherapeutic relationship or to discuss the doctor's personality trends instead of their own problems. Once this is accomplished, he may bring emphasis to bear upon the fact that acting out hinders or delays discovery and investigation of dissociated and repressed material.

As to the psychiatrist's attitude toward a patient's repeated requests for physical examination, all bodily complaints should be checked by physical examination until their organic or psychosomatic aspects are clarified on the physical side. After this has been done, either by the therapist himself if he feels competent to do so or by a qualified specialist in the field, the patient's requests for further examinations by the therapist should be refused. The origin of such continued requests is either a conscious or an unconscious attempt of the patient to delay the psychotherapeutic work because of exhibitionistic tendencies or a wish to seduce the therapist into sexual activities of which the patient may or may not be aware.

Hypochondriasis may be another reason for a patient's craving for physical examinations. Because of the dynamics of hypochondriacal states, refusal is even more important in this case than it is in the case of exhibitionistic or procrastinatory motivations. Hypochondriasis constitutes the danger of a serious disruption of the patient's interest in overt interpersonal relationships, as it entails the danger of the patient's retreat into somatic self-engulfment.

Incidentally, classical psychoanalysis is opposed to physical examination of patients by their psychiatrists. I believe that, by and large, no harm will be done by a physical examination which is medically indicated if and when the psychiatrist is not self-conscious about the procedure and, of course, if he is not guided by any ulterior motives of his own. Young psychotics who are treated by young doctors of the opposite sex may constitute an exception, because with these people the physical examination may arouse an alarming and disrupting amount of anxiety.

Quite naturally, there will be many psychiatrists who will have to refrain from giving physical examinations because of lack of experience in dealing with somatic disturbances. No pretense to the contrary and no veiling rationalizations should be made to the patient when the psychiatrist asks for the help of a colleague. After all, this is frequently done in other branches of medicine. The consultant should be a specialist in the field in question, and it would be preferable that he be experienced in psychosomatics and hence interested in meaningful collaboration with a psychiatrist (95, 165).*

The outcome of patients' attempts at acting out by falling in love with the therapist and wishing to talk or make love has been

---

* Maurice Levine's book (95) can be highly recommended to these physicians.

extensively discussed in the context of the doctor's role in the psychotherapeutic process (Part I) and of the patients' role in their transference experiences (pp. 97–107). The reasons for the incompatibility and the strict technical inadvisability of the consummation of love and sex experiences in the psychotherapeutic setting have also been clarified in this chapter.

The discouragement of love experiences of any mode or description between psychiatrists and their patients for alleged therapeutic purposes is not only a matter of technical rules and regulations. There are two potent reasons of a very simply human nature which make love-making and psychotherapy incompatible. The psychiatrist is not a statue, but a creature of flesh and blood. Therefore, he may wish to make love for therapeutic reasons only, but he may respond to the physical aspects of love-making, in spite of himself, as a person and not as a doctor. Should he, on the other hand, invite or not refuse love-making on the part of the patient without evidencing the physical reactions of a human partner with glandular equipment, he might harm his patient even more, because this would be a demonstration of the patient's impotence in arousing him, i.e., of inferiority as a sex partner.

## 2. HOW TO INTERPRET

Before completing the discussion of *what* to interpret by taking up special mental operations, such as slips, dreams, and hallucinatory experiences, some further general interpretive suggestions should be offered. They will also be applicable to the interpretive approach to these special operations. These suggestions are: first, how to offer interpretations; second, the process of "working through" interpretively clarified material; third, the timing of interpretive intervention.

I shall begin with the problem of *how* to interpret. Respect for the complexity of the patients' collaboration in all interpretive endeavors should color and direct all of the therapist's interpretive activities. To repeat in this context what was mentioned in Part I, the psychiatrist should never feel as if he were a clever detective outwitting the culprit in a simple maneuver. Instead, he should make a point of instigating the patient's interest in cleverly discovering for himself the hidden meaning of his intricate communications. In addition to the respect conveyed to the patient by using this technique, there is another reason for its recommendation. Any interpretation which a patient is able to unearth for himself is more impressive to him, hence more likely to produce an immediate and lasting curative effect, than any interpretation offered by the therapist. This type of approach, by implication, also has the function of assisting patients to gain a greater sense of managing and directing their own lives instead of having their lives directed for them. If the psychiatrist finds it necessary to offer an interpretation, he should always do it in such a way that the interpretation invites further elaboration and does not close the issue under discussion.

Again I wish to offer a clinical example in illustration of these suggestions which stems from the psychotherapeutic experience with a patient who has been previously mentioned in another context (70). A patient was about to be dismissed from the hospital. She was to continue with ambulatory treatment. Two weeks prior to the date set for her discharge, the patient went to the municipal hospital, where she made arrangements to be admitted for a short period of observation. She knew that this was quite in order for people who wanted an unbiased decision about hospitalization, when there was disagreement with relatives or doctors about the need for it. Her expectation about the decision was that it would result in her being pronounced healthy. However, at the last minute she changed her mind and returned to her hospital. Breathless and flushed, she appeared on the dot for her scheduled appointment with her psychiatrist, related the experience to him, and added the following report. She had thought that she actually wished to remain at the municipal hospital for observation, but, at the last minute, when the admitting doctor went to telephone her hospital, she found herself unable to go through with it.

It would have been easy enough for the psychiatrist to point out to the patient that her behavior was indicative of her "ambivalence"; but this merely descriptive interpretation would have been obvious and therefore meaningless. Also, it would surely have closed the issue for further interpretive investigation of the incident. Instead, an effort had to be made to ask an interpretive question that would open the way for the patient to discover the dynamic reasons for her ambivalence. Yet the psychiatrist did not at first know the cause of the patient's display of ambivalence; hence he was at a loss regarding a useful correct interpretive question. He therefore told the patient that he needed a few minutes to think this over. He admitted that, offhand, he did not know the meaning of her behavior or what it was supposed to convey. The patient did not at all resent the psychiatrist's admission that he needed time to consider what the meaning of her behavior was and what it conveyed to both of them.

This, then, is an illustration pointing toward a confirmation of the statement made in Part I, where it was suggested that the psychiatrist would not lose caste in the eyes of his patients if he confessed his need for extra time to mull over their problems.

After further consideration the psychiatrist felt reasonably certain that he understood the motivating factors for the patient's action. Here was a patient who knew that she was soon going to be dismissed from the hospital and that subsequent ambulatory treatment had already been planned for her. Yet, knowing this, she had gone to another hospital with the complaint that she was being forced to remain hospitalized. This was at the point when her own psychiatrist considered her well enough to continue treatment as an out-patient. Therefore, she might well have been successful in impressing upon the physicians at the municipal hospital, who did not know her background, that she was completely cured and in no further need of treatment. Could this conceivably be what she wanted, and, if so, why? If it were the question of further treatment, then the patient's ambivalence must be due to her being afraid of recovery. What else could it be? He then asked her why she was so afraid of an actual ultimate recovery. The patient's response was to burst into tears and say with great feeling, "Are you surprised that I am afraid of actually getting well and having to return to live among my family and friends? Remember that, while I have spent eight years in mental hospitals, they have been in contact with the whole outside world. They have gone through school and college, seen new movies and plays; some of them are married and have children. They have followed political developments and all that sort of thing."

The patient's outburst gave the psychiatrist an opportunity to point out to her that while she had been hospitalized she had gained a far greater amount of experience and knowledge as to what goes on within and between people than any of her relatives or friends. After all, had she not studied and observed the emotional reactions of and the interplay between herself, fellow-patients, nurses, and doctors? The patient was startled, she stopped crying and said with a note of happy relief in her voice, "Hmmm? So it is all a matter of having the courage to look at things from the other side of the fence?"

After that the patient's interest in therapeutic collaboration was renewed. Had the descriptive interpretation of ambivalence been allowed to close the issue—had the patient's own ultimate interpretive conclusion been offered by the psychiatrist instead of the patient's being given the chance to find it herself in response to the physician's pertinent interpretive question, the therapeutic usefulness of this incident would have been greatly diminished, if not eliminated.

This example also demonstrates two more suggestions about the method of the interpretive approach. The first is connected with the psychiatrist's statement to the patient that her psychological experiences in the hospital were a worth-while equivalent to those of her friends on the outside. This response of the therapist was in line with my introductory remarks that there are marked assets concomitant to, or engendered by, the liabilities of mental patients. The second suggestion is demonstrated by the psychiatrist's avoidance of the error of minimizing the emotional significance of the patient's experience, by making a thoughtless remark or by phrasing his question in a devaluating way, as we psychiatrists are so easily apt to do. He might have said, "Oh, this is just your fear of further treatment." Instead of devaluating his question, he stated it with sufficient earnestness that the patient, too, could respond in the spirit of a therapeutically valid endeavor.

Incidentally, this patient touched on a serious problem which is quite common with many mental patients who have been hospitalized for a long period of time. For obvious reasons many of them are slow in adjusting to living on the outside after their dismissal from the hospital, and therefore careful guidance of these patients is recommended for the initial period. Counseling with the relatives, either by the therapist or by a well-trained psychiatric social worker who has been in contact with the patient, may be helpful in the case of some patients (cf. Initial Interview, pp. 45–68).

In the instance of the patient to whom I just referred, posthospital guidance by the psychotherapist was offered but rejected. She accepted the offer of the doctor's contacting one friendly significant relative as perhaps being of some use to her, but she evidenced little enthusiasm for the idea, making it obvious that she wished independently to put to practical use what she had learned.

One more comment must be added here about the possible danger of the psychiatrist's depreciating a patient's communications and experiences, the imminence of which was present but fortunately avoided, as we saw in the case of this patient. Sometimes patients themselves try to induce the psychiatrist to make light of their communications. A statement fraught with implications may be made and then followed by the remark, "That's it, and that is all there is to it." The psychiatrist must cast aside the character of resistance of such a remark. He must also control his own mounting annoyance and avoid the trap of complying with the patient's attempt at eliminating serious consideration of the implications of his communications. In order to do this, he may, for instance, open the discussion of these implications by a remark of this type: "Could it be that in addition to what you said . . . ?"

A patient, for example, may complain about the authoritative, domineering behavior of his boss, which bothers him unduly. He may add, "Why talk about it? After all you can't do anything about it. What's more, it isn't so important anyway." The psychiatrist may feel that it is indicated for him to point out to the patient that his surplus resentment about the behavior of his boss springs from previous anger engendered by his father's domination. Here it is again recommended that the psychiatrist not convey his interpretation by saying, "Oh, that is only because you have transferred your old hatred against your father to your boss." Instead, one might seriously comment that the unduly strong reaction to the present experience may be understood as a result of its being a compilation of the patient's actual plus his transferred resentment. It would not be wise, either, for the psychiatrist to say in a more or less authoritative way, as we are so easily prone to do: "This means that. ..." This formulation may fail to convey to the patient the psychiatrist's expectation of the patient's collaborating with him in the spirit of mutual equality. If, instead, the psychiatrist will introduce his interpretive suggestions with something on the order of: "Do I hear you tell me that ... ?" or some similar remark, he then addresses himself to a psychotherapeutic co-worker, as it were, and so, by implication, invites further interpretive collaboration on the patient's part.

If an interpretation has been found which proves to be meaningful to both the patient and the psychiatrist, the latter must safeguard against the danger of accepting it as final and of closing the issue. The possibility can never be excluded that the psychological truth just discovered may be only partial, so that it is the responsibility of the psychiatrist to be on the alert for changes or additions which might have to be brought forth by further investigation of the same issue.

Incidentally, the patient's affirmation of the correctness of an interpretation by merely saying "Yes" or giving another noncommital sign of agreement, cannot always be accepted as valid evidence of real insight. Agreement is expressed by some patients when they intellectually understand the interpretation offered, in advance of their ability to make it actually a constructive experience of their own. Others may seemingly agree as a means of perfunctory acquiescence. This is true for all types of patients, but especially for schizoid personalities and schizophrenics, who wish to keep the psychiatrist from interfering with their state of withdrawal.

The following conversation is taken from a conventional state hospital case history and offers an illustration of the misleading instigation of meaningless yes-responses by the psychiatrist and for its misleading usage by the patient.

Doctor's question: How do you feel?
Patient's answer: Very well, thank you.
Q: Are you angry with someone?
A: No, I'm not.
Q: Perhaps you are and would not like to talk about it?
A: Perhaps I am.
Q: Are you angry because you are here in the hospital?

A: Yes, I am.
Q: Who are you angry with—mother, father?
A: Yes, I am.
Q: Is it mother?
A: Yes.
Q: Do you dislike mother?
A: Yes.
Q: Father?
A: Yes.

The psychiatrist can be sure that his interpretation is actually meaningful to the patient only if the patient shows by his attitude, gestures, facial expression, or tone of voice accompanying his "Yes" that he has really caught on, or if he confirms an interpretive suggestion of the psychiatrist by a genuinely relevant response or by pertinent associations.

The danger of the psychiatrist's failing to recognize when an interpretation has uncovered only part of the truth is especially great in the case of interpretation of psychosomatic symptomatology. The well-known connections between some emotional and physical aspects of certain syndromes may reduce the psychiatrist's alertness in spotting a patient's additional emotional difficulties which do not find immediate expression in his bodily symptoms.

For instance, take a patient suffering from gastric ulcers and, as their emotional concomitant, from an unrecognized need and longing for dependence (cf. 18, 22, 163, and *Journal of Psychosomatic Medicine*). This patient may develop further emotional symptoms unconsciously aimed at the maintenance and pursuit of his dependent needs. These symptoms may be indicative of unrecognized hatred against those who deny fulfilment of his quest for dependence, or they may be unconscious tendencies to invalid himself in order to become a legitimate object of nursing care. The psychiatrist who listens to the patient with his attention focused only on the equation *ulcer = dependence* may fail to see and to clarify for the patient these additional aspects of his emotional symptomatology.

When the psychopathological aspects of physical ailments were first rediscovered at the beginning of this century, psychiatrists were inclined to oversimplify the possibility of their interpretive comprehension in yet another direction. They tried to understand the emotional significance of physical symptomatology in terms of its descriptive appearance rather than by investigating its dynamic emotional meaning in terms of the somatic etiology of the physical symptom. To put it differently: the development of interpretive understanding and technique of "the language of the body" has followed the same course as interpretation of verbalized communications. However, content interpretation of verbalized manifestations was not relinquished because of its incorrectness but because of its therapeutic ineffectiveness. Interpretation regarding the appearance of bodily manifestations had to be abandoned, though. because this was frequently incorrect.*

Needless to say, the appreciation of the psychosomatic nature of any syndrome should not interfere with a thorough examination of its physical aspects before and, if necessary, while its emotional aspects are being investigated and treated by the psychiatrist (see also p. 78). I believe that one may safely say that there are no physical symptoms without emotional concomitants and no mental disorders without somatic concomitants or causes. At the present state of medical knowledge it is often possible to uncover only the one or the other element in pathological processes. Frequently, the somatic *and* psychological constituents of a pathological process are known. In these cases the choice between somatic treatment and psychotherapy depends upon the decision of which method will be more effective. In this book on intensive psychotherapy we, of course, are referring to psychosomatic syndromes which are subject to psychotherapy.

Two more suggestions about the formulation of interpretations should be added. The psychiatrist should not be afraid to present correct and valid interpretations with the authority of a well-trained person who is certain that he knows his business. His formulations should be short, simply and plainly meaningful, and in the vein of matter-of-fact suggested leads offered by one person, the therapist, to another human being, the patient, who needs guidance. Preachments and recitals are ill advised. The psychia-

* The interpretive approach to the psychosomatic aspects of migraine headaches which I have suggested is an illustration of this viewpoint (61; see also 22). For further literature on this subject see Ref. 171. Wolff disagrees with the hypothesis offered about the psychogenesis of migraine headaches. For further study of psychosomatic problems see Refs. 22, 23, 73, 75, 76, 77, 81, 163, 165.

trist may like the sound of his own voice, but the patient, as a rule, will sense that recitals halt psychotherapeutic collaboration and progress.

The formulations which the psychiatrist uses with each patient should vary according to the type of personality, the particular psychopathology, and the special background of the patient in question. The meaning of thoughts, actions, and feelings in various people, hence also in various patients, is subject to specific modifications. These will depend upon the history and the background of each personality and the respective frame of reference of interpersonal experiences. This will hold true irrespective of certain basic connotations which may be common to the reactions of quite a number of patients with a similar psychopathology. Unless the psychiatrist gears his formulations to these variables, there is the danger that they may be experienced as theoretical or as too abstract or too much like expressions coming "from page 2" of the psychiatric textbook. This will add to the difficulty of a patient's acceptance of an interpretive suggestion per se. Also it will certainly unnecessarily interfere with the transformation of the patient's intellectual understanding of an interpretation into therapeutically effective insight. However, adapting the psychiatrist's formulations to the needs of the patient should not be accomplished at too great a sacrifice of his specific ways of self-expression which, after all, emanate from his own background and personality.

In the case of patients who persist in a refractory attitude toward verbalized routine interpretive work or in the case of an emergency, the psychiatrist should use his ingenuity to expedite the situation. He must call upon those devices which are available to him in accordance with his skill and experience and which are contingent upon his own and his patient's personalities.

In this connection I am reminded of the following illustrative experience. A woman patient who for years had suffered from bilateral trigeminal neuralgias had finally decided on surgical intervention upon neurological advice. One week prior to the scheduled date for her operation the patient came to see the psychiatrist because of pressure exerted upon her by her brother, who was a former patient of the psychiatrist.

In the first interview the psychiatrist cautiously substantiated the idea as suggested by the brother that it might be worth while to consider the possibility of psychosomatic aspects of the patient's symptomatology. A prolonged interview followed, in which information was gathered about the patient's personal and environmental history, about her present life and life-circumstances, and about previous and present complaints. The patient was the eldest of a family of nine. The heads of the family had been a headstrong, but unskilled and powerless, mother and a weak and ineffective father. This made the patient the designated parental guide and adviser of her eight younger siblings. Under the patient's guidance and against her father's advice, she and her sisters got an adequate academic education and social training. Her sisters married in due time and settled down as useful citizens in various walks of life. The only brother was a problem child, who later ran into great emotional difficulties which brought him ultimately into psychoanalytic treatment.

The patient herself had remained unmarried. She had consummated several unhappy love affairs. Professionally she had served successfully in significant positions at various social agencies. When she came to see the psychiatrist, she held a position of importance, ethically and financially, as a leading member of a significant social organization. Asked about the interpersonal aspects of her work, the patient burst into bitter complaints, quite out of keeping with her otherwise very reserved attitude toward the doctor. She complained that her male colleagues did not treat her with the esteem and consideration due her. They did not really take her contributions as seriously as they should be taken in view of her age, experience, and skill. However, factual reports about the patient's working days, the nature of her work, and the collaboration with the men in her organization gave the patient's verbose and tearful complaints a false ring.

Guided by her history and the fallacious reasoning of her present complaints, the psychiatrist suggested the following possibility: Could it be that the patient's complaints about the disrespectful attitude and behavior of her colleagues were a projection of her own attitude toward them? Were painful distortions of the expressive facial musculature one of the patient's means of concealing from herself and others her attitude of disdain of and her sense of superiority over the men in her past and present life? Were these efforts at concealing her real feelings responsible for her facial neuralgias? Here she was: the daughter of a weak, despised father, the sister of a troubled neurotic brother; a girl endowed with the role of a father to her sisters; a self-made woman whose life was marked by a successful career and by the absence of durable relationships with men. Was all this not sufficient reason for and evidence of her feeling disdainful of men?

The patient denied this interpretive suggestion with an amount of vehemence which gave her away in the eyes of the psychiatrist (see "Timing of Interpretations," p. 150). But in several subsequent sessions no awareness for this fact could be promoted in her. Finally, the psychiatrist asked the patient to recall Leonardo da Vinci's portrait of Mona Lisa, with its enigmatic expression of a mixture of female devotion and a smiling sense of knowing superiority which some women feel for men. The patient looked puzzled. A reproduction of the portrait was put in front of her. Upon looking at it, the patient herself put on a Mona Lisa smile. Then she began to weep softly and ultimately accepted the above-mentioned interpretation and the possibility that her trigeminal pain was due to her constant unrealized effort to keep her facial musculature from expressing the sense of superiority, if not of disdain, which she felt for men in general and especially for those with whom she worked.

This happened on the eve of the day for which the patient's operation was scheduled. Early the next morning she called the psychiatrist to tell her that she had canceled the operation and that for the first time in years she felt free from pain. The beneficial outcome of that first two weeks of treatment was reinforced by subsequent psychotherapy. Then the patient moved to another town and another position. In the course of the following years she had some mild relapses of her neuralgia and returned for various short periods of treatment.

This example does not stand, of course, as a representation of intensive psychotherapy as it has been defined in the Introduction. It merely exemplifies the use of a nonverbal interpretive adjunct in the state of the emergency which was created by this patient's pending operation.

We cannot leave the topic of how to interpret without commenting upon periods of silence, with which the patient may present a serious problem to the therapist. Needless to say, silence is frequently hostile and often a sign of resistance or intentional blocking. However, there are also patients who may be silent, because in their early lives there was such a lack of experience in communication that they are at a loss as to how to go about the business of communicating. Other patients remain silent at times because they trust the psychotherapist. He may be the first person in their lives who has presented them with the gift of a degree of interpersonal security which makes it unnecessary for them to speak. These patients are people who in their previous interpersonal experiences have been conditioned to speak not with the idea of communicating but only to cover up their insecurity, like the wanderer who whistles in the dark. In such situations it will be wise for the psychiatrist to make allowances for extended periods of friendly silence. The happy comment of one patient to such a situation of friendly silence was, "The happiness to dare to breathe and vegetate and just to be, in the presence of another person who does not interfere." This patient was the only son of a very hostile, domineering, and obsessional mother (66). The danger that the doctor's needs for security may interfere with his freedom in giving the patient the peace and relaxation of such temporary silence has been discussed in Part I.

In other patients, silence may be due to their need to take time out to think over the doctor's suggestions or newly acquired views of their problems which were instigated during a therapeutic interview. The psychiatrist certainly does not wish to interfere with this kind of constructive silence either. There might perhaps be danger of his doing so, were he motivated by a wrong obsessional concept of the required amount of material which must be covered during one therapeutic interview.

Patients whose silence is motivated by their helplessness in communication or those whose silence is motivated by hostility against the therapist or by reluctance to work on traumatic material need the doctor's help in breaking through their silence. I do not believe, as some psychiatrists do, that there is anything to be gained by the therapist's allegedly waiting until these patients are able to resume verbalized communication by themselves. I consider this to be most unrewarding. First of all, the doctor's silence may easily lend itself to the interpretation of being—and sometimes may actually represent—a sign of *his* helplessness or of *his* hostility. That, of course, will be harmful to the patient, who seeks help and guidance. Furthermore, the loss of time incurred by meeting the helpless silence of a patient by countersilence may be all the more unconstructive because a wall of unending silence may erect itself in these helpless, hostile, or resistive inarticulate patients unless they are given help in an early stage of such periods of unconstructive silence. The various therapeutic devices previously mentioned in other connections have to be used at the discretion of each therapist with each patient, to break through these futile silences.

Prolonged periods of silence in psychotherapeutic work with psychotics constitute another problem in interpretive psychotherapy. The doctor may try to break through the silence of these psychotics by pondering aloud about its possible reasons or by offering some pertinent interpretive remark regarding the emotional material that was under therapeutic investigation before the patients became silent. Above all, the psychiatrist should safeguard against interpreting patients' friendly silence as an attack against his security. He should concentrate his thinking on the patients and their possible needs in order to be alert to any changes in their posture, gestures, or facial expressions which may be offered as an opening for their return to verbalized therapeutic interchange.

I saw one patient for nine months, during which time he was mute except for the utterance of four sentences at the beginning of this period regarding the dynamic reasons for his present apathy and silence. During each interview I made at least one sympathetic remark or an interpretive comment upon the dynamics of one of these four sentences. I tried to keep my thinking concentrated on the patient and the therapeutic problem that he presented. I also attempted to express by my whole attitude that I was with the patient and fully prepared to see him through this period of apathetic silence, until he finally broke through it to resume verbalized psychotherapeutic exchange, which eventually led to his recovery.

Some psychotics are silent or mute because of their hallucinatory preoccupations. In these cases, questioning statements by the doctor—based on guesses, if necessary—may sometimes be the lesser evil as compared with the perpetuation of silence. The patients' gestures, attitudes, expressive movements, on the one hand, and the doctor's knowledge of the general dynamics working in the respective types of patients, on the other, may have to guide him in his attempt to break through silences which appear to be unconstructive.

With neurotic patients, the psychiatrist may also frequently be guided by their inadvertent attitudes, gestures, and expressive movements (19). The encouragement of [mute] patients to draw and to paint is another device successfully utilized by C. G. Jung and his followers and also by the late W. Wittenberg, by Therese Merzbach, and others. The encouragement of patients' humming and singing tunes which they hear inwardly can also be recommended.

### a) THE PROCESS OF "WORKING THROUGH"

From what I have said so far about interpretation, it could appear as though one single interpretive clarification of the origin of a symptom or of an interpersonal problem would have the effect of change and cure, if it were rationally well understood and clarified. Yet the intellectual understanding of an interpretation is not at all identical with a therapeutically valid grasp of its meaning.

Even if the transformation of intellectual understanding into a living emotional acceptance of some piece of interpretive clarification has been successfully accomplished, this generally will still not constitute change and recovery. The reader may recall the general remarks on interpretation on pages 80 ff. and the examples of patients' experiences in point which have been mentioned on pages 105 and 121. As a rule, patients are unable actually to integrate therapeutically effective understanding after one such interpretation of one isolated experience. Furthermore, the pretense or assumption on the part of the psychiatrist or the patient that intellectual understanding due to one single interpretation may help is a dangerous block against real change and real cure.

The question then arises: If access to awareness of dissociated material is a step toward mental health, why does one single interpretation, as a rule, not lead to curative integration of the new understanding? The human mind does not operate, as we know, in terms of independent mental processes; that is, its operating cannot be understood as the sum total of mental operation A plus mental operations B and C. The individual mental or emotional experiences which the psychiatrist and the patient must investigate and interpret, of necessity, in seeming isolation, as they are presented to the therapist's observation, are, of course, part of the person's pattern of reacting and thinking, but they are interlocked with one another in multiple ways. Interpretive dissolution and understanding of some specific piece of dissociated material, therefore, can produce only a certain degree of actual change. The extent to which any single piece of awareness and understanding affects a patient's many other known or dissociated interpersonal experiences, which are mutually interlocked with the first one and through them with his general patterns of reacting and thinking, will determine the extent of real change.

As a result, any understanding, any new piece of awareness which has been gained by interpretive clarification, has to be reconquered and tested time and again in new connections and contacts with other interlocking experiences, which may or may not have to be subsequently approached interpretively in their own right. That is the process to which psychoanalysts refer when speaking of the necessity of repeatedly "working through" the emotional experiences for the dynamics and contents of which awareness and understanding have been achieved, and when they speak of "working through" the elements which operated in the process of establishing this awareness and this understanding (31, 37, 50, 72, 99, 107, 147).*

There may be some readers who may wonder why, so far, I have used only the terms "understanding" and "awareness" and not the word "insight" for the understanding which is accomplished by interpretive clarification. The reason is the following: I wished to convey, by this very choice of terminology, that the intellectual and rational grasp of one interpretation of a single experience, as a

---

* G. Groddeck makes a most worth-while, though purposely not scientific, contribution to the understanding of the process (see Ref. 75). See also E. Hutchinson, Ref. 86. Further literature references are given by these authors.

rule, will be changed only by the process of "working through" into the type of integrated creative understanding which deserves to be termed "insight" (pp. 80 ff.).

The process of "working through" is aimed, then, at changing awareness and rational understanding of the unknown motivations and implications of any singled-out experience into creative, that is, therapeutically effective, insight. This is accomplished by investigating the specific experience which is under interpretive scrutiny per se and in its interlocking ramifications with other experiences. Gaining this type of insight should be accompanied by understanding the previously unrevealed causes for the curtailment and inhibition in the development of a patient's inherent capacities and potentialities. The recall of the first early incidents which were responsible for the loss of the patient's own concepts of his constructive interpersonal capacities plays an important role in the process of the reconstruction of his belief in and of the actual development of his previously eliminated capacities for self-realization and constructive interpersonal relationships.* The actual character of the experience of creative "insight" into, versus the rational understanding of, an interpretation is as difficult, if not as impossible, to define as is the nature of creative processes at large at the present state of psychological knowledge. That was why Freud despaired of coming nearer to it than by describing it as "Aha-Erlebnis," an experience of "Oh, that is it!"

In the course of the working-through processes, special interpretive attention must be paid to the repetitive occurrence of patterns of feelings, thoughts, actions, and behavior, which are dynamically conditioned by one and the same underlying experience which was previously dissociated or repressed. This holds true especially for the repeatedly mentioned four areas of interpersonal experience, toward whose clarification the psychotherapist's attention should be mainly directed: present emotional difficulties in living, developmental history and general biographical data, previous and recent situations of personal crisis, and the vicissitudes of the doctor-patient relationship. Yet even the evidence of the previously un-

* Dr. David Rioch has recently succeeded in promoting significant change in the treatment of neurotics and psychotics by stressing this investigation of the origin of their lost concept of these capacities in their early developmental histories.

known motivation of such repetitive patterns in these four areas of interpersonal experience will not produce change and cure in response to being pointed out and seen just once with the help of the therapist.

For instance, take the woman about whom I reported on page 104, who came to see the psychiatrist following her fourth unhappy love experience. She learned to understand clearly from the psychiatrist's interpretation that her personal attitude toward her parents, her psychiatrist, and her lovers all followed the same pattern of a dichotomy between hero-worship and submissiveness, on the one hand, and the display of a marked sense of superiority, on the other. She also learned to recall the dissociated childhood experiences which were responsible for the development of this pattern. She was made to see that the pattern repeated itself in her presenting problems and in situations of personal crisis evolving from it, her last unsuccessful love experience, which made her decide to consult a psychiatrist. Yet, in spite of understanding this, the patient was *not* able to integrate this knowledge constructively or to change her pattern solely by virtue of the interpretation, recall, and intellectual understanding of the underlying experiences. The childhood experience, its patterning influence, and her intellectual understanding of it had to be worked through repeatedly in its reflections on the doctor-patient relationship and in various other contexts, before the patient's understanding of it was converted into real insight with curative effectiveness.

The patient who became disturbed by the initial interpretive discovery of the possessive nature of her interpersonal attachments may also be recalled in this connection. She spontaneously recognized the necessity of repeatedly working through this new insight in order to make it therapeutically effective (pp. 105–6).

There is one more issue of great psychotherapeutic significance implicit in the discovery of the basic pattern of the difficulties of these two patients which were in the direct focus of psychotherapeutic attention. This issue of the central dynamics of patients' difficulties will be discussed in the next section.

In order to evaluate how much understanding of and insight into his interpersonal processes a patient has gained at a given time, reviews of the material presented and interpreted so far may be given by the patient or by the doctor at regular intervals. These reviews will also help in the appraisal of the general progress of a patient. Further therapeutic help may be effected by inviting corrections and suggestions on the part of the patient to the doctor's review and vice versa. Discussion of the causes and the nature of omissions, additions, or distortions which may appear in these reviews and the patients' own progress appraisal at times will open up new significant therapeutic avenues. In other cases these reviews may prove to be good signposts for the subsequent conduct of the psychotherapeutic procedure.

Working through has a connotation additional to the one upon which I have elaborated so far. In the course of working through the newly acquired understanding and insight, patients should be trained as a matter of therapeutic routine always to test such insight by investigating it in its relatedness to their practical living and to the conduct of their relationships with others. In order that they may do so effectively, the therapist may be required to add to the patients' gain from interpretive psychotherapy by formulating for and evaluating with them the facts and data which in each case constitute their existing testing ground. Because of this, psychoanalysts at times refer to analytic psychotherapy as a kind of "re-education" (see also 3). This clarification frequently forms a valuable frame of reference for the patients' insight into the functioning of their inner minds as well as for their correct orientation in and adequate adjustment to the world outside themselves. Furthermore, the mutual establishment between doctor and patient of a common-sense understanding of universally valid life-realities frequently may help patients to accept new insights which were not accessible to them prior to the doctor's orienting remarks. If these facts and data are presented with intuitive skill and in a matter-of-fact way, for the purpose of patients' practical orientation, they form a significant adjunct to interpretive psychotherapy.

From a host of facts of this type I offer two simple examples: giving sex information to misinformed adolescents and adults, as in the case of the patient mentioned on page 181; or presenting common-sense data about the officially monogamous character of our culture to men or women who pride themselves upon successfully maintaining a neurotic triangle situation in an exhibitionistic fashion.

Sometimes it may be helpful to do more than just to soberly give pertinent information. My efforts in this direction in the case of a young schizophrenic girl may serve as an illustration. This girl had obtained gross misinformation not only about the facts of life but also about the role of women and men's relationship with them.

We had done the required analytic investigation and clarification of the unconscious concomitants of her distorted reactions to the type of information with which she had been misled. After that, she still thought of the menstrual period as "the curse." I offered the suggestion that it could well be thought of and referred to as a friendly "visitor," bringing her monthly messages from her inner organs with their potentially child-bearing capacity. I went on to speak very simply about the asset of natural productivity, etc. Following this discussion I leaned toward her, cupped my hands around my mouth and whispered, "And I'll tell you a secret—delivery is not only painful but can be also both lustful and enjoyable!" The patient replied that she had wondered about that, and upon her return to the ward she spread the exciting news to a friend. Subsequently, both the patient and her friend ceased to have the menstrual cramps from which they had previously suffered.

With the exception of giving this sort of information, the backbone of all intensive psychoanalytically oriented psychotherapy is the correct application of interpretive psychotherapy as it is described in this book.

## b) THE CENTRAL DYNAMICS OF THE PATIENT'S DIFFICULTIES

The interpretive discovery of a common denominator in a patient's pathogenic and pathological experiences has been described in the preceding section. An attempt to achieve this type of discovery should always be in the focus of psychotherapeutic endeavor. This may furnish the answer to the all-important psychotherapeutic question: Which are the central dynamics of the patient's difficulties? When the central problem is found, "working through" should mean that the investigation of whatever is presented by the patient should be conducted in the direction of further clarification of the central dynamics of his difficulties.

Side issues may present themselves at random. At times they come up as resistance against focusing attention on the central problems. As a rule, these side issues can be neglected if and when the therapist is reasonably sure of seeing the patient's central problem correctly. The reason for working through along the lines of the central problems rather than paying attention to all side issues, if, when, and as soon as one really knows the central issues, is the following: As these issues are clarified, minor side issues may yield automatically. Also, patients who are not shackled by the lack of realization or understanding of their central difficulties will be able to recognize and handle the side issues under their own steam.

To illustrate: a patient who was suffering from severe obsessional symptoms and phobias could not walk unaided from my office to her home, over a long period of time. Suddenly one day, while still under treatment, she found herself doing so, to her utter amazement. We did not find out, therefore, through which channel of ramifications this symptom had been reached therapeutically, before it subsided. Incidentally, the patient, being an obsessional, was quite unhappy to lose a symptom without knowing why. The therapist, however, could not be induced to waste time on the investigation of this specific issue. She preferred to accept the fact that the symptom had yielded in the course of the general therapeutic procedure. Eventually, the patient accepted this therapeutic attitude. The fact that there was no relapse helped her to do so.

This patient did recover and has remained well for the last fifteen years without ever gaining special interpretive insight into the specific reasons for the loss of one of her symptoms. The clarification of these symptoms was not mandatory for the understanding of the central dynamics of the patient's difficulties.

To repeat then: it should depend upon the usefulness for further clarification whether content material which patients produce after the doctor has recognized the central dynamics of the patient's difficulties may be included in, or discarded from, interpretive attention. The only area of investigation for which this does not hold true is the investigation of the vicissitudes of the doctor-patient relationship, which has to remain in the focus of psychotherapeutic attention throughout the course of the treatment.

My suggestion of concentrating psychotherapeutically on the central dynamics of a patient's difficulties as soon as one knows them is not intended to advocate that a patient who may need intermediary steps should be indiscriminately rushed into concentrating on central issues before he is actually able to do so. It is the doctor as the participant observer in the psychotherapeutic procedure who must constantly keep in mind the central issues in patients' psychopathology while listening to them and while conducting psychotherapeutic procedures.

Psychotic people, especially, often cannot be rushed into concentrating at a set time on central issues which they themselves do not yet have in mind. Severe states of panic and anxiety may be elicited under too heavy therapeutic pressure. The psychiatrist should also remember that in the mind of many psychotics the experience of the time element involved differs markedly from his own (cf. pp. xiii and 167).

Neurotic patients who work with unnecessary delay may be successfully pushed toward more speed in their productions and in their attempts at interpretive understanding of the central dynamics of their difficulties. As previously mentioned, the therapist will not harm them in doing so if it is done for the patients' benefit and not to satisfy the therapist's ambition. As a rule, anxiety will not grow beyond the limits of the endurance of psychoneurotic patients, and the sense of time by which their lives are governed coincides with that of the psychiatrist. Therefore, he does not run up against these unknown entities in his efforts to speed up the tempo of their psychotherapeutic collaboration.

Of course, neither do I mean that, while working through the patient's productions, guided by his central dynamics, the psychiatrist should listen while prejudiced by his preconceived ideas about the patient's problems. The contrary should be true. The psychiatrist should watch and listen with vigilant care and alertness for any possibility of the patient's uncovering new slants on the dynamics of his difficulties. While listening, he should, at one and the same time, connect what he hears with the central difficulties, as he sees them at the time, and check on the correctness of his view.

The following is an excerpt from the treatment history of a patient in whose case it was comparatively easy to focus upon the central dynamics of his difficulties. The presentation of these relatively uncomplicated central dynamics should not mislead the psychiatrist into underestimating the difficulty of getting central problems crystallized in more complex situations. But it may help to sensitize the reader's alertness to the possibilities of this part of the psychotherapeutic process.

A brilliant, efficient, and successful professional person came to see the psychiatrist. The primary complaint was that he felt very anxious and ill at ease with other people and that he suffered from unexplained phases of fatigue and exhaustion. He reported a great number of incidents which were all analogous, including the last one, which caused him to seek psychotherapeutic help. The patient was only partially aware of this. His complaints were that he could not assert himself, could not ask for what was rightly due him professionally or personally, and could not fight back when he was hurt or verbally assaulted. Here is an account given by a man who was successful in his profession and well liked generally, although with no intimate relationships. Each of his experiences evidenced a disconcerting lack of self-assertiveness. He feared that he might lose his job if he talked back to his boss. He was afraid that his associates might resent his participation in an argument with any of them, irrespective of whether he was right or wrong regarding the issues discussed. He was fearful of losing caste in the eyes of a friend of his if he merely requested the friend's child not to touch some of his beloved gadgets. He was haunted by the fear of threatening repudiation by and isolation from his family, should he offer the slightest disagreement. This feeling existed despite his being a well-appreciated and adequate, though cautious, provider and despite the fact that the various members of the family bestowed upon him all the signs of acceptance and respect for which he yearned. In brief, when not working or sleeping, this man spent his life propitiating people and "keeping under control" all self-assertive tendencies. He had to do so because he felt perpetually haunted by the fear of impending disaster. These were the words used by the patient himself while describing in detail several of the above-mentioned incidents.

Needless to say, the patient repeated this pattern time and again in his dealings with the psychiatrist, without realizing its repetitional character. Unknown to himself, this patient was obviously frightened of repressed impulses of hostility and destructiveness. That was why he spent his life placating and propitiating everyone with whom he came into contact. Because of lack of data, the

*What about Shame?*

nature and intensity of the hostile impulses could not be brought home to the patient for a long time. Finally, it appeared that the patient had "forgotten" to mention a brother, four years his junior, when giving his family history. This brother had lost one leg during World War II. The patient held himself responsible for this war casualty, even though he had in no way been instrumental in his brother's joining the armed forces, much less in his being sent to the combat theater where he was wounded.

These data furnished the psychiatrist with the knowledge of the patient's wishes for his brother's death and of the patient's belief in the magic power of his wishes. He felt responsible for his brother's being maimed because he wanted this to happen to his brother. The patient was then guided by the psychiatrist's interpretive questions toward uncovering himself, his envy and hatred of his brother, and his destructive impulses against him. They had originated in an early phase of the patient's developmental history, when the childhood belief in his omnipotence was still operating and when there was only a very dim awareness of the difference between thought and action. This childhood relationship with his brother, which was perpetuated outside awareness and therefore never revaluated, was the primary root of the patient's anxiety. As soon as psychiatrist and patient could see this clearly, the patient could also learn to understand that, unknown to himself, all his interpersonal dealings were governed by destructive tendencies and by regressive fantasies regarding his omnipotence and the magic power of his hostile, destructive thoughts and wishes. Also without being aware of it, he felt so threatened by these fantasies and the concomitant anxiety that something in him expected them to come into the open and to become effective whenever he found himself in the slightest disagreement with another person, whether it was his brother, the psychiatrist, or anyone else. Therefore, he had to spend his life in self-control and propitiation and in a constant state of fatigue and exhaustion. He had to expend too much energy to keep in check his unidentified destructive impulses and the anxiety aroused by them.

Thus a central problem of the patient could be focused. The same problem had been in operation in his early childhood in his relationship with his brother. It also repeated itself in the acute situation of distress which brought the patient into psychotherapy, as well as in all his previous and recent interpersonal relationships and in his interchange with the psychiatrist. When this central problem was brought into focus by the psychiatrist and recognized by the patient, the working-through of pertinent data and their interpretive understanding could be guided in the direction of gaining lasting experiential, hence ultimately curative, insight into the genetics and the central dynamics of the patient's psychopathology.

## 3. TIMING OF INTERPRETATIONS

This completes the comments upon how to interpret and what to interpret, and I shall continue now with the discussion of the timing of interpretations. The same suggestions which have been offered regarding the formulation of interpretations also stand, *mutatis mutandis*, for their timing. As a rule, interpretive suggestions or questions should not be offered unless one has at least an over-all picture of the personality and the basic psychopathology of the patient to whom one offers the interpretation. The question of how to go about obtaining such a picture has been discussed in the chapter on "The Initial Interview" (p. 45). It is true that there are many types of reactions outside a patient's awareness which are so generally human or so generally characteristic of a specific type of psychopathology that their meaning, although hidden from the patient, may be understood by the psychiatrist without further knowledge of that person. Yet, as a rule, it is wise to refrain from evidencing such understanding before one is able to operate on the basis of an approximate knowledge of the background and personality of the patient with whom one is dealing. This rule does not apply to open manifestations of resistance and security operations. As previously discussed (pp. 107 ff.), it is good therapeutic technique with most patients to point these out as they occur.

The following are some general considerations which the psychiatrist should have in mind while deciding about the correct timing of his interpretations. The reader will see that practically no rules can be suggested without enumerating the indications for exceptions. It must be left to the experience and the intuition of the psychiatrist to decide when to follow the rules or when to make use of suggested exceptions.

As soon as a workable doctor-patient relationship has been established and as soon as the psychiatrist approximately knows with whom he is dealing, he should be ready, in principle, to approach his patients with active therapeutic moves. The fact that they may not be able to accept them immediately is not necessarily a sign that the approach is counterindicated. The suggestions offered may have to be repeated, and their results may have to be worked through innumerable times, but that should only rarely be a reason for refraining altogether from therapeutic intervention.

This suggestion is not intended to exclude the possibility of establishing a therapeutically valid relationship with a patient by offering interpretive reactions to his manifestations. In the hands of a skilled and experienced person who is not afraid of the hostile outbursts with which some patients may respond, favorable time-saving results may be obtained with the use of this technique. The doctor must also be sure that his interference is not prompted by unwarranted "countertransference" but solely by therapeutic considerations.*

If a patient gets upset or angry about an interpretation, this is usually indicative of its being correct or at least in the immediate neighborhood of correctness. Otherwise the patient would not react so strongly to the interpretation. Hence it follows that patients' outbursts of anger, etc., in response to interpretations are no contraindication against pursuing them. As a rule, the contrary is true.

Marked glibness or blankness in response to an offered interpretation is indicative of its being doomed to therapeutic ineffectiveness for the time being, i.e., it is ill timed and working on it should be postponed.

As a rule, it will be wise to offer interpretations and to try to elicit interpretive responses from a patient after he has reached a stage bordering upon an awareness of the subject of interpretation. It is then that the psychiatrist may be most successful in conveying

* Dr. Mary J. White, of the Chestnut Lodge Sanitarium, has recently been able to demonstrate this. The similarity to and difference between this approach and Rosen's may be noted (see notes pp. 95 and 180).

to patients the experience of discovering their final interpretations by themselves, as was recommended in the discussion of the question of how to interpret. This suggestion should not be followed, however, at the expense of directness and spontaneity in the doctor's attitude.

Again, generally speaking, interpretations should be offered only if and when all data pertinent to the issue under interpretive investigation appear to be covered by the interpretation and if the psychiatrist feels reasonably certain that the interpretation he has in mind is the one which he considers correct and valid among several other possibilities. It may be indicated, though, that this suggestion should not be followed in the case of patients whose therapeutic interviews lag markedly and are unproductive. If and when this situation fails to be remedied over a period of time, then stirring up and stimulating acceptance or refutation of the doctor's interpretive suggestions may be the one valid way to promote fruitful psychotherapeutic exchange. Also in such cases it may be indicated sometimes that interpretive suggestions be given prematurely, that is, before their validity is fully corroborated. The therapist must then be prepared to run the risk of having his suggestions prove to be subject to later correction. By and large, patients will be not harmed but helped by the occasional usage of the device of a thoughtfully directed "shot in the dark." Needless to say, I am not advocating the use of random interpretations but of suggestions which quite likely will be correct. Their validity, however, may not be beyond question and may depend upon further proof.

There are two more points determining the correct timing for interpretive procedures which were mentioned in the discussion of the interpretation of resistance. These also hold true for the interpretive approach to all other issues. First, there is more hope for successful therapeutic utilization of interpretations, offered or elicited by the psychiatrist, if this is done while the patient's relationship with the psychiatrist is a predominantly friendly one in its real and in its parataxic aspects. Of course, clarification of the hostile aspects of the relationship per se at times constitutes an exception to this rule (cf. pp. 107–18). Second, the patient should be able to handle the amount of anxiety which the psychiatrist expects to be released by his interpretations, without developing serious additional symptoms during the interval between two interviews.

Of course, in the case of hospitalized patients, the need for caution regarding the release of anxiety is less than with ambulatory patients because psychiatric help is available if and when the patients' anxiety warrants it. In the case of psychoneurotic patients with marked hysterical trends, the therapeutic release of anxiety is not too dangerous as a rule either. In fact, the contrary is frequently true. The tension aroused in these patients by certain interpretations may force them into resuming therapeutic collaboration to an extent to which they were not interested prior to the burdensome rise of anxiety. In interpretive work with disturbed psychotics, especially schizophrenics, the slowed-down, narrowed, concrete thought-processes and the specific time conceptions of the patients will have to be especially considered in timing rational interpretations. (For further suggestions regarding differences in the interpretive approach of various types of patients see the general introductory remarks, pp. 80–84.)

I remember in this connection the disturbed schizophrenic about whom I wrote in a previous publication (66). His progress seemed so exceedingly slow to me that at times I asked myself whether there was any progress at all or whether I was handling him incorrectly and should transfer him to a colleague who might be able to be useful to the patient in a shorter time. One day this patient commented spontaneously, "Things are going surprisingly well between us except that they are going too fast. If only you wouldn't rush me so that I would not have to go so rapidly."

A psychoneurotic patient may express a similar type of reluctance to responding to therapeutic suggestions in line with the doctor's tempo. In his case, however, this reaction would be promoted by the fear or anxiety elicited by the therapeutic intervention. Time must yield to his needs, and quite often the neurotic in fantasy succeeds in misinterpreting or in changing the passage of time in accordance with his wishes. The schizophrenic patient's quoted response was dictated by the inherent difference between his attitude toward chronological time concepts and those of the mentally stable (pp. xiii, 147, 167). Psychotherapists must remember this difference in patients' attitudes toward time and timing while deciding about when to offer therapeutic intervention.

## 4. INTERPRETATION OF SPECIAL
## MENTAL OPERATIONS

### *a*) SLIPS AND ERRORS

The discussion about the application of interpretations will now be continued with some remarks on the interpretive attitude of the psychiatrist toward special mental operations which he will encounter in the course of the psychotherapeutic process. These are the slips and errors of everyday life; the daydreams and the dreams of the sleeper as they are presented by both neurotics and psychotics; and the hallucinations, delusions, and persecutory ideas of psychotics.

First, we shall investigate the usefulness for interpretive psychotherapy of the slips and errors of everyday life. They are, as we know, such phenomena as forgetting; mislaying; errors in printing, writing, and reading; being too late or too early for an appointment; stumbling over someone's feet; running into someone; etc. Freud taught psychiatrists to understand all these phenomena as products of a compromise between intentions, which are in awareness, and the interference with the intended act by dissociated or repressed impulses, which are not permissible within awareness (49).

Concurrently, then, the validity of the psychoanalytic thesis that all mental manifestations are meaningful also holds true for the slips and errors that occur in people's everyday lives. The fact that their occurrence is markedly facilitated by physiological phenomena does not detract from their psychological significance. All degrees and phases of lowered physiological capacity, illness, exhaustion, and overexertion interfere with the alertness of those parts of the personality which control awareness. Therefore, repressed impulses have a greater opportunity to interfere with the intended acts of overtired persons.

Slips and errors were extensively used in interpretive psychotherapy in the early developmental phase of psychoanalysis. In later years most psychoanalysts altered their views about the psychotherapeutic value of the interpretation of slips. There are a number of reasons for this change of precept. First, there was an increase in the general psychoanalytic knowledge about the vicissitudes of the interaction between tendencies which are dissociated or repressed and intentions which are within awareness. This, of course, made slips and errors less significant as dynamic sources of interpretive investigation than many of the other mental processes which are more characteristic of the patients' interpersonal difficulties and whose interpretive significance we have previously discussed.

Another reason is that the interpretation of slips easily lends itself to the danger of being done as therapeutically disconnected content interpretation. Such a procedure would be in direct contrast to using or encouraging the patient to follow the dynamic and genetic interpretive approach for therapeutic purposes, which has been suggested in the preceding sections.

A third reason for the change is that psychiatrists have learned to see that the slips and errors are not so simply and unilaterally meaningful as was previously thought. What has been suggested regarding the interpretation of other dissociated or repressed phenomena, therefore, also holds true regarding slips: they should be interpreted only, as a rule, when one is sure that all pertinent data are known and covered by the interpretation.

A fourth reason concerns certain dangers which may occur when slips and errors are interpreted indiscriminately. Let me offer a hypothetical case in point. A therapist, proud and gleeful about his secret knowledge of a patient's hidden impulses, jumps at interpretive conclusions about his "telling" slips as they occur in the current psychotherapeutic situation and in the patient's interpersonal dealings with the therapist. He offers his so-called "wisdom" to the patient. In doing so, he may well add unconstructively to a mental patient's ever present burden of self-consciousness. Also he may interfere with the psychotherapeutic build-up of the patient's impaired spontaneity.

The psychiatrist should make an inner note of one or another slip when he first observes it, if the slip appears to furnish an important contribution to the general understanding of the psychopathology of a patient's interpersonal operations. It will then be available for later reference in a constructive context; but by no means should it be employed by the psychiatrist for jumping at premature conclusions and their interpretation for would-be psychotherapeutic use.

Because of the reasons given, forewarning against the general therapeutic use of slips and errors, their interpretive utilization is now recommended only if and when no other usable data are available. In its absence, one or another slip or error may be interpreted if it seems outstandingly conclusive or suitable to demonstrate an unknown impulse to the patient, the exposition of which seems to be therapeutically meaningful at a special point of the treatment.

The interpretive approach to slips is unnecessary in psychotherapy with psychotics, unless a baffled psychotic introduces the subject himself, implying that he wishes the psychiatrist's comments. This, of course, may be deduced from my general remarks about interpretation on pages 80–84, where I have elaborated upon the difference between the dynamic significance of the repressive and dissociative processes in psychotics and neurotics.

As an illustrative summary of the remarks on the interpretive significance of slips and errors, I wish to offer an example of a misinterpretation in my own experience. A patient who had his analytic appointment at night after the termination of his working hours had been five minutes late for each of his interviews. For many months the psychiatrist did not comment on this apparently repetitive slip. However, she made a mental note about the necessity of discussing it with the patient, sometime soon, as an indication of his negative transference or resistance.

Fortunately, the patient volunteered his own information before the psychiatrist had an opportunity to offer her incorrect interpretive assumption. He told the doctor that he always arrived at her office in time but that he felt like waiting five minutes before coming in, in order to give the doctor a respite of five minutes between patients. There was no maid or secretary there at that time of the evening, so it was necessary for the doctor to answer the door herself; the patient wished to spare the doctor this interference with her privacy during the interval between two interviews. There was no reason to question the correctness and sincerity of the patient's information, hence of the incorrectness of the interpretive slant of the psychiatrist on the patient's alleged slip.

The question then arose: Was this action of the patient really what it was intended to be, that is, an act of well-planned consideration; or were possessive elements at work in the patient's attempt to run the doctor's schedule more favorably than, in his judgment, she seemed to be able to do herself? In other words, the patient's action first presented itself to the psychiatrist as a plain slip, obviously determined by dissociated negative impulses against the psychiatrist and the patient's work with her. Instead, it turned out to be within the patient's awareness—an intended act of considerateness. Unknown to him at the time it was first discussed, it appeared to be the result of a possessive and domineering attitude toward the psychiatrist. This latter interpretation could be corroborated in the further course of the treatment. This example then illustrates the multiplicity of possible causes for an action which presented itself at first glance as a plain slip which seemed to lend itself to one obvious interpretation.*

## b) DAYDREAMS

Daydreams, that is, a person's private reveries and fantasies, are the next type of mental operation which I wish to discuss with regard to their significance in interpretive psychotherapy. Daydreams are covert, "prototaxic" (147), autistic, interpersonal thought-processes—reveries, fantasies—which are concerned with the satisfaction and security of the daydreamer. Actual reality is disregarded, the course of events in the outside world is imaginatively rearranged in the dreamer's thinking to fit in with his personal fantasies. Therefore, daydreams are an important source of material from which the doctor and the patient may acquaint themselves with the hidden contents of the patient's thinking and feeling, particularly with his desires for fulfilment and self-realization.

In this culture there is a predilection for daydreaming during the period of adolescence. What happens then represents the function of all daydreaming throughout life. Adolescence is the time

---

* I am indebted to Dr. Karl Menninger for his contribution to the interpretive understanding of this patient's "slip."

when adult ways of fulfilment of one's goals of satisfaction and security may be anticipated in daydreams. It is only later that the psychobiological and educational equipment for their attainment is accomplished, and the social modes of our culture permit the teen-ager actually to experiment with reality in seeking satisfaction and security. As the healthy adolescent matures and finds the fulfilment in reality of what he has anticipated in his daydreams, his reveries will more or less diminish or disappear.

An adolescent's dream about a fairhaired, blue-eyed princess may be his initial quest for the prototype of the girl whom he will court in the future. This dream girl may or may not be like his childhood recollection of his mother or his sister; likewise his choice of her may or may not be determined by his rebellion against the attachment to some significant females of his early life. Irrespective of these genetic considerations, her image may be indicative of what he will look for in reality later, unless his visionary picture of her is so conventionalized through the influence of screen, comics, pinup girls, or fiction that she is not representative of his own actual choice and taste. If the daydream of his beautiful blonde princess is really self-determined, it may bring to fruition his search for a girl with whom he can ultimately share what the adult man wishes to share with his partner: love, sex, and intimacy.

The daydreams of another teen-ager about his professional or business career may be the cradle of his actual choice of job or professional training in the future. Just as he loses himself in adolescent reverie and dreams about philosophy, peace, change in the order of the world by evolution or rebellion, just so this may later determine his career as politician, newspaperman, member of the diplomatic service, the army, or the navy, etc. And again, looking at it from the genetic viewpoint, this dream may or may not be influenced by the juvenile or preadolescent image of his father or brother, favorite uncle or influential teacher.

We see the same operation at work in the adolescent who revels in seemingly masochistic daydreams about being bitterly wronged by his father, teacher, or superior and who indulges in expansive fantasies about how "to get even with" them and how "to show" them. This may be the expression of alarming neurotic tendencies in this boy, but it may also be the adolescent psychological predecessors to the boy's learning to defeat fear and anxiety and to brace himself for adult self-assertion in the future.

The degree of daydreaming in later life will generally correspond to the amount of interference and frustration which a person has had to contend with in the pursuit of his goals of satisfaction and security. As just mentioned, it is similarly determined in adolescence by the discrepancy between the conception of the desired goals and the psychobiological or sociological interference with their immediate attainment.

Of course, it is of the greatest therapeutic significance to detect the unconstructive escapist elements in and the hidden meaning of a person's daydreams and to help patients to understand the first and to dissolve the latter. However, there is danger in being too quick on the trigger with interpretation and devaluation of the constructive significance which the daydreams of mature people may have in common with many of the reveries in adolescents.

The daydreams of creative people have been recognized as one of the significant sources of art production ever since psychoanalytic attention has been directed to people's reveries (94, 113, 124, 153). Tension caused by the discrepancy between actual and wished-for fulfilments in a person's life may sometimes be discharged when the artistically creative daydreamer is able to interpolate his conflict into the lives of people of his own creation.

From what has been said it follows that daydreams and their creative transformations can function as preventive mental hygiene for the dreamer. Frequently this also holds true for the daydreams of noncreative people, who keep them in their private reverie world. Their daydreams may furnish temporary substitutes for the frustrating aspects of their actual lives, which otherwise may lead to the development of emotional disturbances.

Psychiatrists have not paid enough attention to this aspect of daydreaming. Most of us became too preoccupied with the quality of unreality in the daydreams of our patients and hence overestimated their need for active intervention by the therapist in the role of a watchful denizen of outward reality. We were either so busy training patients to do more adequate reality testing or so occupied in trying to find out retrospectively what people or what events were forebears of the patients' daydreams that we neglected to explore sufficiently the question of mental hygiene and the prospective significance of daydreams. The daydreams of any one of us today may well represent our anticipated accomplishments of tomorrow.

Because of this, daydreams are among the most cherished private mental processes of the mentally stable and of the mentally disturbed. If they lend themselves to interpretive investigation at all, it is usually only after a patient's treatment has been under way for quite some time. If a patient finally relates his daydreams, the psychiatrist, as a rule, should consider this to be a distinct sign of trustful psychotherapeutic collaboration. Hence he should handle the daydreams of his patients with gentle care. He should never fail to consider their wishful fantasies as a valid source of information about their real problems. To repeat: He should, of course, pay serious attention to their possible use for unconstructive withdrawal from reality; but he should abstain from entertaining the preconceived idea that all daydreams are necessarily due to a nonconstructive flight from reality; he should try to listen attentively to the constructive lead which is frequently involved.

Of course, there are also patients whose daydreams have a predominantly escapist, hence unhealthy, character, just as there are a few adolescents who sometimes lose themselves in the confusing maze of their daydreams. This modicum of patients needs psychotherapeutic help in order to learn to recognize the quality of and the reasons for the disturbing unreality of their daydreams. This does not mean that they always call for direct interpretive intervention in their own right. They may frequently be used to greater therapeutic advantage as additional material when the developmental history of the patient and the dynamics of his other problems are worked through, and, as a rule, it should be possible to resolve them in this connection. In most cases when direct interpretation is attempted, the rule should be followed more than in any other field of interpretive psychotherapy that interpretation should be preceded by ample informative questioning designed to encourage the patient's further sharing of his private thought-processes with the therapist. By the mere process of relating and thus sharing them, they are changed from covert to overt interpersonal processes. Following the release of daydreams from the patient's private inner world, most patients automatically take care of their own reality testing.

With all patients it is indicated that the psychiatrist offer repeated warnings against confounding dreams and fulfilled accomplishments. This is intended to serve as a safeguard against patients' taking the doctor's therapeutic interest in the constructive aspects of their daydreams as an encouragement to daydream rather than to work toward the fulfilment of their reveries in the real outward world. After these warnings have been given and heard, many patients may need help only in realizing the constructive aspects of their reveries. They may not have been able to see this constructive aspect because of the guilt feelings which frequently accompany daydreaming.

The mixture of this alleged sinfulness and embarrassment may frequently account for the patient's guilt feelings, which may arise from the fantasied superiority of the daydreamer or from the self-centered character of his dreams or from the effortless gains about which he daydreams. Often, however, they are not instituted by the contents of the daydreams. They stem from the very nature of its privacy, since the significant adults of the dreamer's childhood were originally excluded from sharing his reveries. Remember, parents are supposed to know everything about the child, just as the Lord does. This feeling is expressive of the widely accepted tenet that children are the spiritual possessions of the parents, just as the parents and the child are the possession of the Lord. Therefore, it may be considered sinful to withhold daydreams from the knowledge of one's parents.

### c) DREAMS

In continuing the discussion of the interpretation of special mental operations, I shall now take up the interpretive attitude toward the dreams of the sleeper. If the reader will recall my introductory remarks about the similarity between dreams and psychotic productions, it will facilitate his understanding of this chapter.

Dreams present the thoughts, feelings, and hallucinated actions which a person experiences while asleep. Being asleep means having withdrawn one's awareness from the world and one's interest from any happenings which do not concern one personally. Therefore, the dreamer's thoughts, feelings, and hallucinated actions are mental manifestations operating during states of eliminated or markedly reduced awareness. Hence they are not submitted to the control or censorship which regulates the manifestations of a (nonpsychotic) person while he is awake and aware of actual happenings inside and outside himself. The censorship of the ego is off guard (119), the critical control of the self as custodian of awareness is eliminated (147). The mental manifestations of the dreamer are not geared to the necessity of adapting to environmental standards, and they are not colored by the need to strive for or to maintain one's position among one's fellow-men (59). Because of this, the dreams of patients offer an important means of understanding their actual modes of thinking and feeling. Therefore, dream interpretation is used as an integral part of psychoanalytic psychotherapy.

It has been repeatedly mentioned that strict precautions be used in employing any of the interpretive techniques discussed in this book. Their use, as mentioned in the Preface, is intended only for psychiatrists who have undergone thorough training in the application of these techniques and who, through their own didactic psychoanalysis, have gained insight into their functioning. Special warning must be given here against the unskilled use of dream interpretation. It should not be used by anyone, therapeutically or otherwise, unless he is thoroughly familiar with its technique and with all its implications.

The brief discussion of dream interpretation which I shall subsequently offer is not designed to teach the reader how to interpret dreams for therapeutic purposes. At best, it is intended to outline the basic principles of therapeutic dream interpretation. Those who are interested in learning how to apply it therapeutically must do so under expert guidance by studying the extensive literature and by repeatedly attending classes, seminars, and group discussions on dream interpretation (31, 52, 72, 99, 123, 139).*

The interpretive attitude toward dreams and their psychotherapeutic usefulness should be determined by the psychiatrist's realization of the state of mind of a dreamer during sleep and by his

---

* See also extensive literature in the *International Journal of Psycho-Analysis, Psychoanalytic Quarterly*, and *Psychoanalytic Review*.

knowledge of the mental operations and the means of expression specific to the mental condition of the sleeper.

It is equally important, however, that a psychiatrist know the person whose dream he is to interpret and that he be acquainted with the person's history and life-experience. He should also know approximately the setting in which the dreamer lives at the time of dreaming and of presenting his dream. This holds true for the problems of dream interpretation, just as it does for the psychiatrist's general interpretive attitude, as previously recommended.

What must a psychiatrist know about the dynamics of dream processes? Freud has mentioned most of them in his epochal work on dream interpretation. A great many of his conceptions still hold their place as the cornerstones of therapeutic dream interpretation. Every dream reflects the impression of events in the dreamer's life which have happened either the day before the dream or some days previously. While awake, the dreamer may, or quite frequently may not, have been aware of the psychological importance of these events per se or of their relatedness to other events of equal or similar emotional validity in his past or present life. In addition, there will always be reflections or direct representations of the patient's present conflict or crises situations. Therefore, one way of using dreams for psychotherapeutic purposes is to bring these events and their representations and reflections to the dreamer's recognition or to increase his awareness for them in connection with his dreams.

Another therapeutically helpful means of gaining access to the actual thoughts and feelings of a patient, through his dreams, is the following: while under intensive psychotherapy, dreams are frequently used by the sleeper as a means of conveying something to the therapist which the patient has been incapable of conveying while awake. All the other implications in the doctor-patient relationship which have been discussed throughout this book may also be reflected or represented in the dreams of every patient under treatment. According to Gittelson (112), a direct, undistorted representation of the therapist in the dreams of a patient may indicate the dreamer's realization of the therapist's countertransference difficulties.

One more avenue of approach to the sleeper's interpersonal experiences that is opened by the dream gives access to childhood memories. In people's waking life the engrammatic and patterning influence of these memories is frequently shown only by implication. In most dreams, however, childhood experiences are directly repeated (see also the section on "The Initial Interview," pp. 54–55).

The psychiatrist not only must be familiar with these facts but must also know the modes of operation and the "language" which the dreamer uses to express his thoughts, feelings, and hallucinated actions, in order to be able to interpret patients' dreams and to guide them in their attempts at doing so themselves. The means of expression used by the sleeper are those which are characteristic of people in states of eliminated or reduced awareness. A knowledge of these means of expression and alertness in understanding them are prerequisites for the understanding and interpretation of dreams. That is, this knowledge gives access to the latent, real meaning of the manifest dream contents as presented by the dreamer. This statement does not imply that one knows how to interpret dreams if one knows the language of the dream, it only implies that one is *not* able to understand and interpret dreams if one does *not* know the specific language of the dreamer (144).

With this warning in mind, we can now proceed to enumerate the means of expression characteristic of dream processes. First, the dreamer uses imagery rather than spoken words. For instance, a writer finds himself faced with a seemingly insuperable obstacle in the formulation of a difficult philosophical problem. He may express this experience in a dream by seeing himself on the bank of a river which he should cross in order to complete a difficult journey. To cross it appears impossible, since the current is swift and there is no bridge (140).

The second way in which the dreamer expresses himself is by symbols and pictures. I shall offer elucidation of this by giving some suggestions offered by Freud within the frame of reference of his interpretive approach to dreams as sexual wish-fulfilments. Freud says that sticks, canes, or snakes may stand for the male organ and that holes and openings may represent the vagina. Houses, churches, and ships may be used as maternal symbols signifying the womb; airplanes and birds, which rise against the laws of gravity, may symbolize men or the male organ. While these symbolisms are true for some patients and for some dreams, one must be very cautious in safeguarding against acting under the presupposition of the universal validity of these or any other symbols. Their significance definitely varies with the personality, the life-circumstances, and the problems of the dreamer. In one person's dream, for instance, a snake may appear as a male symbol, while another dreamer may use a snake to express female shrewdness and seductiveness. Again a snake may be used by an archeologist to express the attributes of one or another of the multitude of male and female gods or goddesses whose total or partial embodiment is that of a snake (88). Special symbolic significance must be attributed to numbers (52, 78). Where direct verbalizations are used, as a rule they are repetitions of verbalized exchanges of preceding days. Most of the time they are verbatim as originally spoken. Verbs, i.e., expressions of action, as a rule, are more helpful clues to the understanding of the latent meaning of a dream than are nouns.

Third, the dreamer expresses himself in allusions, and he experiences delusions and hallucinations, as in the following dream fragment. A dreamer is concerned with an important emotional experience which took place when he was five years old. He neither sees nor thinks of himself at that age but sees the house where a five-year-old niece of his now lives. While dreaming this, he hallucinates the smell of the cake baked for his fifth birthday, and he sees the niece's house and smells the odor of the birthday cake. In the dream he finds himself in his present study, and his studio couch is covered with a bedspread which his parents used when he was five years old. This dream fragment is not only illustrative of the dreamer's use of allusions (dreamer when he was five: five-year-old niece) and hallucinations (the smell of the birthday cake) but also of some further modes of operation. They are condensations, distortions, displacements, and interchange of people or objects of similar emotional validity. The couch in the dreamer's present studio covered with his parents' bedspread is a product of such a condensation.

An additional example which at the same time shows the dreamer's interchange of people is offered in the dream of a patient who had suffered from parental neglect when a child and who was concerned in his dream with the longing for the love of a maternal person. He dreamed about a white-haired woman who was wearing a green apron and black slippers. The white-haired woman reminded him of a benign aunt; the green apron identified the gardener, who was a benevolent companion in his childhood years; the black slippers were worn by the cook, who was the only person who came to look after him at night when she heard him cry.

Another characteristic feature of the mental operations in dreams which has been mentioned in the Introduction is that they do not follow the logical syntactic rules governing thought and speech in waking states. They follow the rules of regressive, autistic mental operations—"prototaxic" and "parataxic" operations, in Sullivan's language. Their logic is the "logic" of infants, primitives, or psychotics. It should also be noted that there is no logical connection between various dream elements and that there are no conjunctive parts. The sequence of various dream parts is distorted as compared with their actual logical sequence.

Emphasis may be by repetition of the same contents in various contexts and connections. These repetitions may occur within one or several dreams dreamed in one night or in several dreams dreamed in subsequent nights. This is exemplified by the above-quoted dreams of the patient who evidenced a threefold repetition of his concern about an experience which happened in his fifth year. This shows also in the two biblical dreams of Joseph, which will be quoted later.

There is another characteristic feature of dream expression which is an outcome of the fact that dream expression does not follow the logical rules of mental operations in waking states. In dreams many experiences, thoughts, and feelings are expressed in concepts which are diametrically opposed to what is actually meant. For instance, privacy may be signified by a large crowd, secret knowledge of a document by many people reading it, etc.

There is no logical sense of time and space in the dreamer's mind. Concepts of chronological time or of space in a topographical sense are neglected or confounded. We saw this done by the dreamer who expressed the same experience in terms of his five-year-old niece's present home, the cake baked for his own fifth birthday, his present studio couch, and a bedspread he remembered from his childhood days. The same type of operation can frequently be observed in psychotics. To them, as to the dreamer, a span of years or miles may be condensed into two minutes of experience. Conversely, the dreamer may feel, after having dreamed only two minutes, that he has covered a span of many years or miles.*

Silberer and Tausk were able to demonstrate that some of these means of expression are used even before people are really asleep and actually dreaming. That is, they may be used in the state of incipient withdrawal of interest from and semi-awareness of the outside world, which is interposed between states of wakefulness and sleep (140, 153).

There are two excellent extraneous ways of becoming acquainted with and sensitized to the language of the dreamer. One is furnished by studying the means of expression as they are used in the productions of psychotics (see p. 86). The other extensive source from which one may become familiar with the dreamer's modes of expression is furnished by folklore, fairy tales, and legends, in which dreams are recorded which people have had in common throughout the centuries (125, 140).† Frequently, the author or authors who created them may have been as unaware of their actual meaning as the audience who enjoyed them. Then, again, the meaning of some legendary dreams may have been quite evident to the authors who created them and to their contemporary readers, whereas their "language" needs translation as the language of the dreamer does, in order for it to be understood by the average audience of this era and culture. Yet these tales owe their popularity to their esoteric meaning, just as people's great interest in dreams has its origin in the realization of their hidden meaning. The story of "Sleeping Beauty" is as good an example as any of the popular fairy tales to illustrate their similarity in means of expression with those used by the sleeper in his dreams (131). On her thirteenth birthday, Sleeping Beauty makes a forbidden visit to her grandmother in a distant part of her father's castle and inflicts a bleeding

* Differences between the therapeutic use of dream interpretation with neurotics and psychotics still have to be developed, pending further scientific investigation.

† Jung is foremost among the authors who have pointed out and done research on this subject. As an example, see Refs. 90 and 170.

wound on herself by pricking her finger with her grandmother's distaff. Right after that, the young princess and the whole castle fall asleep until her prince reaches her by breaking through the hedge of thorny rosebushes which have grown around the castle, to find her and to marry her. To translate: at the age of thirteen Sleeping Beauty begins to menstruate, and she is indoctrinated in the facts of life by an older woman, her grandmother. However, she remains an unawakened female until the male partner opens the hedge (the hymen) which has separated the young virgin from her self-realization as a woman.

Another source from which the therapist may increase his familiarity with the language of the dreamer, in addition to studying his own dreams and those of his patients, are the dreams and their interpretations which are to be found in the Bible, in drama, poetry, and fiction from ancient times to the present. The classic Greek dramatic literature and the plays of Shakespeare are especially fine sources for this material.*

The Bible calls to mind the dreamer Joseph, who expresses his superiority over his parents and his eleven male siblings by imagery in the dream that the sun and the moon, his parents, and eleven stars, his siblings, bow to him. He emphasizes the significance of the contents of this dream by repeating it in a second dream in which the sheaves gathered by his brothers are bent down in the fields, in marked contrast to those which he has gathered and which stand erect. The Bible relates that Joseph's dream came true, thus establishing it as a prophetic dream, as he became the chief counselor of the Egyptian Paraoh and, as such, greatly superior to his parents and his siblings (cf. Mann, *Joseph the Provider* [New York: Knopf, 1948]).

As we know, prophetic dreams play a great role among biblical stories; in legends, poetry, and fiction; in lay literature on dreams; and in the minds of many dreamers, both patients and nonpatients. The possibility of increased clearness and astuteness in the thinking of the dreamer, owing to his withdrawal from the distracting and

---

* See, e.g., Romeo's dream in *Romeo and Juliet*, Act V, Scene 1; Gloucester's dream in *Henry VI, Part II*, Act I, Scene 2; Caesar's dream in *Julius Caesar*, Act II, Scene 2; or the dream of Richard III in Act I, Scene 4, of *Richard III*.

In modern literature Franz Kafka's *The Castle* and *The Trial* are wonderful examples and priceless objects of study, to facilitate the understanding of the modes of expression *in* and the atmosphere of the world *of* the dreamer.

inhibitive influences of his outward environment, may make his appraisal and judgment of any given situation so alert and sharp that valid conclusions with possible applications for the future may sometimes be the outcome.

Quite generally it may be said that, since sleeping eliminates the distracting function of awareness of and interest in the outward world for the sleeper, the mental operations of the sleeper frequently excel in wisdom and insight those which he is capable of accomplishing while awake. Most people have had the experience of solving, while dreaming, problems which seemed to have no solution while they were awake.

The elimination of the interference of the outward world from which the dreamer's interest is withdrawn has one more noteworthy type of influence on the quality of his dream operations. Some patients will be more clever, witty, charming, and given to producing amusing similes and puns in their dreams than in their mental operations while awake, frequently very much to their own and the psychiatrist's surprise.

Freud, who was the father of modern psychotherapeutic dream interpretation, introduced a teleological concept with his hypothesis that most dreams are disguised expressions of wish-fulfilment for the dreamer. According to Freud, most of these wishes are sexual wishes rooted in the dreamer's present life and/or in his childhood. Since they are unacceptable or forbidden in the mind of the dreamer while he is awake, they are accomplished hallucinatorily in dreams. Freud credits this as the reason for the dreamer's use of "the dream language," "the language of the unconscious," in his dreams, as a device for disguising the latent dream contents. This will safeguard against the dreamer's realizing the meaning of the dream and therefore against interference with his sleep by the recognition of the hallucinatory fulfilment of these sexual wishes which are culturally or personally forbidden.

The basic assumption which we have offered here is that dreams simply represent what a person thinks and feels or hallucinatorily acts while awareness and censorship are dormant. From this concept it follows that the type of mental operation and the means of expression used by the sleeper in his dreams are explained by the state of reduced awareness of the sleeper per se. Hence it may be seen that these modes of expression will be used by the dreamer, regardless of whether or not the dream content is of a forbidden nature and irrespective of Freud's hypothesis of its teleological motivation. Moreover, it seems to me that there are so many dreams which do not deal with recognizable wish-fulfilments, in the manifest or in the latent contents, that the concept of the universal character of dreams as disguised expressions of fulfilments of unacceptable wishes is open to controversy and revision (52).*

By these statements I do not mean to deny, of course, that there are many dreams which represent past and present, acceptable and prohibited, wish-fulfilments or that there are dreams which deal with sexual thoughts, feelings, and activities in one or all of the various strata of experience which find their representation in patients' dreams (cf. p. 164).

Fulfilments of forbidden and acceptable wishes of all kinds and description, including sexual ones and others, of course, are among the mental productions of the dreamer. Everyone, mental patient and others, is much more freely able to realize his personal longings, ambitions, wishes, and cravings while his thoughts and feelings are not under the censorship of the conventionalized existence of his waking states. Inasmuch as past or present sexual problems and wishes are an important part of the interpersonal experiences in everyone's life, thoughts, feelings, and hallucinatory activities of a sexual nature will, of course, play an integral role in the average person's, hence also the patient's, dream life.

So much for the dreamer's modes of expression with which the psychiatrist should familiarize himself if he wishes to understand and have patients understand their dreams. Doctor and patient should learn to understand dreams in their expression of childhood memories, as they repeat remnants of experiences of the days preceding the dream, especially in regard to present conflict and crisis situations, and as they reflect the patient's relationship with the psychiatrist. This will help to tie these elements together interpretively and thus facilitate the processes of working through and of finding the patient's central problems.†

* See, however, Introduction, p. xiii, about another dynamic teleological significance which may possibly be attributed to dreams.

† Sterba (145) mentions the validity of certain acting-out processes as associations to dreams.

The greatest source of help in this endeavor is the patient's own associations to his dreams. Before a therapist makes any attempt to interpret a patient's dream, the patient should be asked for his associations to the dream as a whole, to its various parts, and to single items in it which seem to warrant special attention. The patient should then give his own viewpoint as to the meaning of the dream. Only when all that the patient has to offer is exhausted, should the therapist step in with his attempts at interpretation.

One exception to this rule may be made in cases in which the therapist or the patient himself feels that the patient is reciting an important and conclusive dream, the immediate therapeutic use of which may throw significant light on hitherto unexplored areas of the patient's interpersonal experiences. In such cases, if the psychiatrist has exhausted the afore-mentioned resources which make dreams therapeutically useful, he may offer what seems to him an interpretation or an interpretive suggestion to the dream as a whole or to certain parts, right then and there. With this incentive in view, the psychiatrist's own interpretive associations may give access to the patient's further interpretive associations. The suggestions of the therapist may be modestly offered for what they are worth, that is, as his associations which may or may not be valid. He should make a point of telling the patient that the final decision about the therapist's interpretive associations lies with the confirmatory or refuting associations of the patient, which the psychiatrist hopes to instigate by offering his own.

Sometimes, when one is doubtful about the meaning of some element of a dream which seems to deserve special attention, it will be wise to ask the patient to repeat the recital of the dream. Those dream parts which undergo a marked change in the second report are deserving of the therapist's special attention. In his attempts to understand them, it may be useful to face the patient with the difference in his two recitals and to invite his associations to this difference.

The question of how much use a therapist should make of dream interpretation with each of his patients depends to a large extent upon the personalities of the doctor and of the patient who are engaged in the psychotherapeutic procedure. Some psychiatrists and some patients are endowed with much talent, while others are less gifted in coping successfully with dream material. Some patients offer enough meaningful general material to fulfil all the purposes of therapeutic investigation and interpretation. In such cases the special interpretation of dream material may not be an addition of great therapeutic significance to the total process of treatment.

In Freud's estimation, dreams furnish the royal road to the understanding of otherwise hidden emotional experiences. With some patients who are good dreamers and poor producers of other material, this holds true magnificently. Other patients may produce unending numbers of dreams during therapeutic inerviews as a means of resisting constructive therapeutic intervention on the part of the doctor. Again, various patients may be capable of producing dreams complying with the alleged expectations of their therapists. Needless to say, these two types of dreams are therapeutically useless as to their contents. They are helpful only for the clarification of the resistive or the compliant aspects of the patient's relationship with the doctor by which these dreams are motivated.

The decision concerning when to use and when to refrain from using therapeutic dream interpretation with a patient should, as a rule, rest in each individual case with the psychiatrist who conducts the psychotherapeutic procedure. Incidentally, he can easily encourage or discourage dreaming or, more correctly, the recall of dreams in most patients, by the degree of attention or inattention which he pays to the recital of their dreams.

The following three types of dreams form an exception to the psychiatrist's freedom to reject or emphasize dream interpretation. The first dream dreamed by a patient under treatment should always be remembered for future reference by the psychiatrist and the patient. The therapist may not understand its meaning when he first hears the dream. It will reveal itself, however, after he has become acquainted with the dreamer and with the genetics and dynamics of part of his difficulties. Frequently, the first dream will then be found to be an expression of a patient's central problem in a nutshell. The second group of dreams which should always be taken into consideration are repetitional dreams which a patient has dreamed throughout his life or which he dreams during the period of treatment. The recommendation that attention be paid to these dreams is self-explanatory. In the case of all patients, dreams in which there is expression of marked emotions and/or marked anxiety, for obvious reasons, should be among those upon which interpretive attention should be focused.

In using dreams for psychotherapeutic purposes, psychiatrists should keep in mind that it is not at all necessary to translate every dream to completion in all its aspects and interpersonal layers. The psychiatrist may have to try to understand all dream parts and the total dream as a contribution to the insight into the one specific part which he has under scrutiny with the patient. As far as the patient is concerned, the interpretation of and the insight into one enlightening aspect of a dream may sometimes do more for him than the time-consuming investigation and interpretation of the dream as a whole and in all its parts. At times it may be even more helpful to use patients' dreams, predominantly or exclusively, for eliciting meaningful associations to the dream material which has not appeared in any other context. They may furnish therapeutically significant clues for further insight into patients' hitherto unknown mental processes and into the dynamisms of their difficulties.

To summarize: The psychiatrist's attitude toward the dreams of his patients should be determined by the patients' therapeutic needs, i.e., by the realization that the therapist's obligations toward the patients are those of a physician and not those of an expert in dream interpretation in its own right.

### *d*) HALLUCINATIONS AND DELUSIONS

Our next topic is the psychotherapeutic approach to hallucinations and delusions. Before speaking about the interpretive attitude of the therapist toward these phenomena, I would like to clarify precisely to what phenomena I refer by these terms. Descriptively speaking, hallucinations are perceptions without sensory foundation in the environment (166). Dynamically speaking, they owe their inception to the bursting-through into awareness of certain dissociated impulses which become so overwhelmingly strong that they cannot be retained in dissociation or smoothly discharged with slight awareness or with none at all. As a result, they express themselves in terms of the noticed autonomous activity of the various modalities of sensation, as subjective visual, auditory, ol-

factory, tactile, or gustatory perceptions without objective foundation. Auditory and visual hallucinations are encountered much
more frequently than the other hallucinatory experiences (147).

If it is true that hallucinations are due to strong repressed or dissociated impulses which burst into awareness, then it follows that
all hallucinations are on the basis of remote or recent real experiences, as in the following case: A young patient had a difficult time
during the Christmas holiday season. Her therapist suggested that
they not skip their interview on Christmas Day. "There he is, the
giant with the ether gun," was the patient's unexpected answer to
the therapist's offer. Asked what she was referring to, the patient
was able to say that the giant and the smell of ether appeared each
time that she was deceived. She was sure, she continued, that the
psychiatrist was deceiving her when he said that he would see her
on Christmas. Such things just did not happen. Asked if she could
remember when being deceived had been linked up for the first
time with the ether gun, she immediately recalled an operation
which had been performed on her at the age of three. She had been
told that it wouldn't be she who would be operated on, but her
doll. Ether was the anesthetic used. The ether was administered
suddenly while she was still expecting to see what was to be done
to her doll. It was as if someone had shot ether at her. Before she
was really under, things and people appeared tremendous, and the
picture of the doctor who operated on her had been retained in her
memory ever since as that of a giant. Here was deception on the
part both of the patient's parents and of the doctor. It was connected with the sudden experience of the smell of ether imposed on
her by a huge man. This, then, was the actual experience which
gave rise to the hallucinatory repetition of the experience which
the patient underwent when she expected to be deceived by the
psychiatrist.

Delusions originate in the realm of thought-processes owing to
the same dynamics which govern the rise of hallucinations in the
sensory apparatus. They are, at least partly, beliefs or interpretations of facts independent of the actual meaning of these facts.
That is, they are false beliefs and false interpretations and exagger-
ations of facts which are the unrecognized expression of repressed
or dissociated material. Hallucinations and delusions are of a strictly

[ 174 ]

psychopathological nature, even though they may occur as fleeting experiences in otherwise nonpsychotic people. Note, therefore, that they cannot be used per se to make a differential diagnosis between neurotic and psychotic disturbances.

Illusions are misinterpretations of actual sensory perceptions, in contradistinction to the perceptions without sensory foundations which we call "hallucinations" (166). Illusions are experiences which may occur in everyone's life and with which we all are familiar. Seeing a tree at night as a person, mistaking moving grass for water or animals in motion, or seeing a stick as a snake are examples of such illusional misinterpretations.

Persecutory ideas are delusions of being persecuted, most of the time, unknown to the patient, because of unacceptable inner impulses. Responsibility and blame for them are passed on to the alleged persecutor. As a rule, these paranoid persecutory ideas are accompanied by delusions of grandeur: one must be a person of great importance to warrant persecution (31, 48).* In a mitigated form the persecutory delusions of the psychotic may be found as transitory ideas of reference in persons suffering from milder mental disorders.

As a general dictum, these three types of mental experience should be submitted to the same principles of interpretive approach as are all other psychotic and neurotic manifestations. The psychiatrist should not argue about their hallucinatory, delusional, or illusionary character. He should state quite simply and clearly that he does not see or hear what the patient professes to see or hear or that he does not share the patient's hallucinatory, delusional, or illusional interpretation or evalution of facts. After that, he should try to interest the patient in the investigation of the following questions: (1) Why does he see or hear what the psychiatrist does not see or hear? Why is there a difference in the patient's evaluation and interpretation of facts and perceptions from those of the psychiatrist and the other people in the patient's environment? (2) Does the patient remember at what time during the psychotherapeutic interview or previous to it the hallucination, delusion, or illusion under investigation first appeared? (3) Can he account

* About Freud's psychoanalytic concept of the origin of paranoia and persecutory ideas see Ref. 48.

for previous real experiences in the remote or recent past which preceded the present hallucinatory, delusional, or illusional experience?

It is true that many psychotic patients will not be able to respond to any of these questions offhand. Also, some of them initially may not even be able to conceive of the questions and their meaning. Even in the case of these patients, it will prove to be useful, however, for later reference to have the verbalized attitude of the psychiatrist on record, as suggested. In addition, many even seriously disturbed psychotics can be trained to observe these dynamic and genetic connections.

The actual experiential background of hallucinations and delusions will frequently be found to be a condensation of various single previous experiences. Much alertness, time, and effort may have to be expended before the historical and dynamic roots of the hallucinatory or delusional experience under scrutiny can eventually be disentangled.

This is demonstrated by the following example: An eighteen-year-old schizophrenic girl complained about severe persecutory ideas, to the effect that she could not bear to have anyone standing or walking behind her. Something frightful would happen to her, perhaps a stab in the back or, at any rate, something terrible, the thought of which made her shudder. She was paralyzed and could hardly move whenever there was someone behind her or whenever she sensed that there might be someone back of her. She did not dare to go downtown because there always seemed to be someone right behind her. Questioned about the actual experience which the patient might consider as the first one of its kind, she said that she could not remember. But she did volunteer the information that, as far back as she could remember, her father had warned her against men who might persecute her and rape her. This happened long before the patient knew what "rape" was and what men might "do" to women. Further investigation of and associations to her fantasies regarding rape and regarding her persecutory delusions disclosed that the form of the patient's persecutory ideas were due neither to her fear of nor to her secret wish for rape only, as one might have easily suspected. Eager to safeguard against therapeutic operations with any partial interpretive truth, the psychiatrist asked for further associative memories to the patient's delusions. The patient recalled eventually that at the time of Hitler's invasion of Czechoslovakia her father had condemned, with great affect, "the stab in the back" done to the Czechs. She was too young to know that father was referring to people and thought he was talking about the checks in the tablecloth on the breakfast table. It was at the breakfast table and while reading the morning paper that her father had these emotional outbursts which were incomprehensible to the patient. Also during breakfast her father would scold the patient severely for various types of infantile misdemeanors about which he had just been told.

Another associative memory came from a later period of the patient's life. Her parents would find out that she had taken money from them, that she had bought hair ribbons or sweets against their wishes, that she had teased her baby brother or the dog, or that she had antagonized the maid. Her father would throw a temper tantrum and say that she was betraying her parents and the training they had given her. The use of the word "betraying" reminded her of her father's using the word "betrayal" in connection with "the stab in the back" to the Czechs.

As a result of a condensation of these memories, the patient experienced her persecutory delusions to the effect that she dreaded that someone behind her would "stab her in the back"—betray her, rape her—as she allegedly had stabbed in the back, that is, betrayed, her parents when she had stolen pocket money or when she had committed any of the other above-mentioned childhood sins. Father had reacted the same way, namely, with a heavy temper outburst, to both types of stabs in the back, hers and the one done by Hitler to the Czechs. Besides, the Czechs had been the "checks" of the tablecloth to her, and father had thrown temper tantrums about her, too, when she misbehaved. So the temper tantrums about the "checks," about her earlier and later childhood sins, together with the fear of rape with which her father had imbued her, were condensed into the patient's formulation of her persecutory delusion of being "stabbed in the back" by someone who was behind her.

What was previously said against the advisability of overemphasis of content interpretation, in general, also holds true for the interpretive attitude toward hallucinations, delusions, and illusions. If patients are not too much under the pressure of the disturbing influence of their hallucinatory and delusional experiences and therefore not too much in need of discussing them, it frequently will be advisable for the psychiatrist to ignore them while working on other important interpersonal experiences. It not infrequently happens that hallucinations and delusions will disappear in the course of the general interpretive psychotherapeutic procedure without having been submitted to direct interpretive endeavor. I have described and discussed the reasons for the disappearance of other symptoms under the same psychotherapeutic regime on pages 127–40. In the case of symptoms of hallucinations and delusions, it is evident from the very definition that was given regarding their dynamics why they may disappear in the course of the interpretive approach to other material. If we assume it to be true that these symptoms are due to the bursting-through into awareness of an unbearable surplus of repressed or dissociated thoughts and feelings, then it is feasible for them to yield when enough material is brought into awareness in the course of the general interpretive process to make unnecessary their uncontrolled breaking-through as hallucinations and delusions.

In this connection I recall the catatonic patient who recovered after eight years of hospitalization and four years of intensive psychotherapy and whom I have repeatedly quoted. She surprised the psychiatrist during an interview which took place about two years after the beginning of her treatment and two years before her dismissal, by making a spontaneous statement to the effect that her hallucinations had gone and that she considered this a marked sign of improvement. Prior to this statement she had only once mentioned that she was hallucinated. At the time that this happened she had been able to accept the therapist's comment about the private and unreal character of her experience along the lines of the suggestions given above. However, she stated frankly that this insight did not do away with the hallucinations, and this comment was accepted by the psychiatrist at its face value. The hallucinations had not been referred to since then by either therapist or patient. It had been obvious, however, that the patient had continued to be hallucinated for some time after this conversation.

This was evident by her marked periods of withdrawal into what appeared to be states of autistic hallucinatory preoccupation. It may be assumed that the psychiatrist's knowledge of the perseverance of her hallucinatory experiences was taken for granted by the patient until she could eventually inform the therapist of their disappearance.

When hallucinations first arise, they usually have a most disturbing and disquieting influence on patients. As time passes, patients learn to adjust to them and to acquiesce. There are rare cases of patients who are under such strong disconcerting pressure from initial hallucinatory experiences or when the disquieting influence may persevere to such a degree that their preoccupation and disquiet interfere with the psychotherapeutic collaboration. The above-described rational approach or interpretive clarification of other topics is, of course, impossible in these instances, and the psychiatrist has to resort to another approach. In these rare cases he may temporarily have to enter as a participant in the hallucinatory or delusional world of the patient.

An example in point is an experience which I have reported before (69). I shall repeat it here in the hope that the experience may be as helpful to some readers as it was to me at the time of its occurrence. A patient was subject to gravely disturbing persecutory delusions night after night. Powerful people of various nationalities were after him. He tried to escape being caught and pleaded with each of the persecutors in his own language. During the day this patient was in rational contact. There was no memory of his nightly delusions and therefore no possibility of discussing them with him. The patient's only complaint was that he could not concentrate and that something interfered with the pursuit of his professional obligations. He did not know what it was except that he felt worn out and beaten down upon awakening in the morning, as though there had been some terribly frightening and trying experience during the night. A number of futile attempts were made to discuss the patient's delusions, about which the psychotherapist had been informed by the nurses' reports. The therapist finally decided to have the nurses awaken her at the time when the nightly delusional experience started, in order to make it possible for her to observe the patient and to participate in his experience. With the therapist present, the patient got up and climbed from his bed to the bureau, from there to the wardrobe, and from there to one piece of furniture after another as though running from his persecutors, pleading with them alternately in English, French, German, and Hebrew. The psychiatrist followed him on his climbing excursion as best she could, trying to reassure him in whatever the language of the moment was by telling him that she did not see the persecutors but that, if and when she caught sight of them, she would try to protect him against them. After about fifteen or twenty minutes the patient quieted down, went to bed, and slept for the rest of the night. The psychiatrist's participation in the delusional experience of the patient had to be repeated once or twice before she was successful in breaking through the wall which the patient had erected against their recall. After that the road was open for the application of the above-described interpretive approach to the patient's persecutory delusions and to the severe states of anxiety which accompanied it. A successful genetic and dynamic interpretive investigation of his persecutory system became possible and in time revealed the nature of the patient's underlying problems. Subsequently, his rational communications could be worked through interpretively in connection with his delusional ideas, and both could be related to these problems. After one and one-half years the patient was free from symptoms and left the hospital and the city where the psychiatrist lived to resume his professional work in his home town.*

* John Rosen in pursuit of his previously quoted method of direct analytic interpretation prefers to use this approach of totally entering into the delusional world of his disturbed schizophrenics (135, 136). For a tentative appraisal of Rosen's therapeutic results see p. 95 n. While comparing Rosen's and this writer's therapeutic techniques, it may be helpful to recall that all mental patients—neurotics and psychotics—are not able to live on the level of their actual chronological age. The psychotic's interpersonal experience and expression is partly on the level of an infant and a child, while at one and the same time there is the body of experience collected through the years which he has lived. Hence one psychotherapeutic problem in working with disturbed psychotics is that the psychiatrist actually must deal constantly with both the infant in the patient and the person of his present chronological age. It may well be that a partial difference between Rosen's technique and the one suggested here is, in the last analysis, more one of degree than one of kind: Rosen addresses himself more to the infant and the child in the psychotic. The method advocated here is based on stressing psychotherapeutic contact with the patient as a person of his present age level (28, 29, 68).

A warning against any attempt to talk patients out of their hallucinatory or delusional experiences by rational explanations or argumentation should be added at this point. It will be doomed to failure. There is only one thing along those lines which at times one may try with hope of success. The psychiatrist can give enlightening explanations of facts and data about which patients were misinformed either in childhood or later, if their misconception of such facts seems to be in part responsible for the contents of the delusion. The patient who feared being stabbed in the back, for instance, was enlightened about the comparatively small percentage of actual cases of rape in comparison with the frequency of the fact as suggested by her father's preoccupation. This plain statement of facts at the end of the interpretive investigation of her delusion seemed to give her some relief.

Incidentally, this patient tried to make sure that the psychiatrist was not just appeasing her but was giving her true information, by asking for further enlightenment about sexual data. In doing so, she wanted to submit the psychiatrist's reliability to a twofold test; she wished to ascertain that the doctor's information would be just as different from father's data as from the romantically falsified enlightenment which she had obtained from her mother. When the psychiatrist passed the test, the patient felt that she could use her relationship with the doctor as a medium through which her experiences in and her hold on the reality of the outward world at large could be revaluated and re-established (see also p. 144).*

* Kempf (91) agrees in many ways with the treatment suggestions given here. Incidentally, the reading of his classical treatment histories is highly recommended. Schilder (138) counteradvises intensive psychoanalytic psychotherapy with disturbed psychotics as useless. For other types of psychotherapeutic approach see Refs. 21, 80, 82, 98, 110, 111, 166, 168.

# CHAPTER IX

## *How To Begin and How To Terminate a Psychotherapeutic Interview*

WE HAVE concluded the discussion of all the elements which constitute the psychotherapeutic process, that is, the material to be offered by the patient and the tools to be used by the psychiatrist. How to handle initial interviews has been discussed, and the problem of terminating treatment will be taken up later. In addition, quite a number of examples were offered to illustrate certain psychotherapeutic operations used in specific situations as they may arise in the course of the treatment. There may still be a question in the minds of some readers, though, about just how a psychiatrist should begin and terminate an interview during treatment.

Many patients will take care of this problem themselves. In the initial interviews they have been initiated into the rudiments of the method of collaborative techniques and into understanding the goal of intensive psychotherapy. After that, any patient who is not too disturbed, blocked, or inhibited to hear the psychiatrist should be taught that, in principle, the responsibility of making good use of the time spent with the psychiatrist by no means rests only with the doctor. The patient is expected to take care of his share by presenting pertinent material for psychotherapeutic discussion, barring his emotional inability to do so.

Frequently a patient will need help in tying up the first communications of an interview with significant experiences on the outside which have immediately preceded the interview or with pertinent contents that were under discussion either in a previous interview or in the last one. If the patient is not immediately able to get started by himself, the psychiatrist should first give him time to collect himself and gradually to begin speaking. He may allow for short periods of silence for this purpose, but he should not wait too long before interfering. The suggestions previously given regarding the psychiatrist's interpretive attitude toward the patient's silence should also be applied with regard to his attitude at the start of the hour.

The psychiatrist may try to help the patient get started by encouraging the investigation and discussion of what prevents the patient's talking or by asking him whether he expects help in getting started. If so, the reasons for this expectation or for this need for help should be discussed. If the patient is not yet ready for this type of therapeutic scrutiny, the psychiatrist should proceed in his attempts to help the patient get started. He may ask him whether his reluctance is due to an immediate or past experience, the recital of which seems difficult, or whether his hesitancy is connected with a difficult or problematical experience which he has undergone in one of the previous interviews. If the latter is true, was this while working through strongly emotionally charged material which came to the patient's awareness at that time, or was it due to some still unclarified real or transference aspects of the doctor-patient relationship?

Some patients may be able to respond favorably to questions of this type, while in others they may arouse a negativistic reaction. With these patients, it may be good technique for the psychiatrist to ponder aloud to himself, either about what he considers to be the likely reasons for the patient's reluctance or about such aspects of the preceding interview or interviews the mention of which, in the psychiatrist's judgment, may presumably arouse a response in the patient and start him communicating.

If the patient himself refers to an experience which he has undergone during a previous interview or to an outside experience which he has previously related, the psychiatrist, of course, is expected to know about it in either case. If he does not, this lends itself to the interpretation that he lacks interest in the patient or in his affairs. Even more harm will be done by pretending to recall, if subsequent remarks do not refresh his memory. The best way to handle this is simply to admit the failure to recall and to express regret. At the same time, the doctor should establish the fact that this is a functional, not an intentional, failure, which at times will be inevitable. The expression of his knowledge of this inevitability should not constitute an excuse for a previous lag in attention on the part of the psychiatrist, who may have drifted away instead of listening. When a psychiatrist is uncertain of his memory, it is advisable for him to take notes following an interview and refresh his memory by reviewing them prior to the next interview with that patient. Because of its disruptive influence on the directness and spontaneity of the doctor-patient relationship, I consider it bad technique, however, to take notes during the interview.

Sometimes the psychiatrist will consider it important that a subject of therapeutic investigation of a previous hour be discussed further. He should try to evaluate at the beginning of the new interview whether the patient is under any special pressure of recent origin which calls for immediate communication. He should also inquire from the patient whether he came prepared to discuss any pressing material which is on his mind. If both these possibilities can be ruled out, the therapist may suggest that there be further discussion of the topic which he has in mind. In other cases he may consider it preferable to wait until an opening for his suggestion presents itself, by the very nature of the present communications of the patient.

In the event that the psychiatrist mentions that it is advisable or necessary for a previous topic to be discussed, he should make certain that this suggestion is followed through and that it is not dropped in the further course of treatment. If he neglects to do so, it may turn out to be discouraging to the patient because it lends itself to the interpretation that the doctor does not place too much value upon his own suggestion. He thereby creates doubts in the patient's mind, either about the professional qualification or the professional self-appreciation of his doctor. The other equally discouraging possibility in the patient's mind may be that the doctor is not sufficiently interested or is so discouraged regarding the outcome of the treatment that he feels it useless to press the issue.

In addition to the previously mentioned starting points, comments upon the patients' appearance, indicating either their emotional and physical well-being or their impairment, and questions about the reasons may help some patients to get started in an interview. If legitimate complaints about physical or emotional symptoms have marked the course of the preceding one or several interviews, inquiry about them may well be indicated at the beginning of the present meeting. This is not recommended, however, if the psychiatrist's inquiry is likely to be misinterpreted by the patient as an encouragement for hypochondriacal preoccupation or for hysterical flight into illness. As a rule, the patient will have evidenced his predisposition to do so prior to the current interview, so that the alert therapist will be forewarned against using this device with patients whom it may harm.

In the case of an inarticulate psychotic, collateral information may be used. Sometimes one may have to use this device also with other types of patients who may know quite well that there were legitimate sources of collateral information. The psychiatrist must be cautious, however, and not put the evaluational judgment of anyone other than the patient or himself upon these data before he has had an opportunity to check on their validity with the patient.

Some psychiatrists may feel called upon to use comments about their observations of the patient at fortuitous, nonprofessional meetings, in order to get an interview off to a start. Caution and discretion should be used in this means of approach. Such comments made by the psychiatrist may easily cause a mental patient to become more self-conscious in his social activities. The necessity for this precaution is self-evident in cases in which repeated meetings are likely to occur, such as at concerts, theater, sporting events, etc.

These suggestions may suffice as a guide for basic orientation on the matter of getting an interview off to a good start. In the same vein, I will now discuss some considerations which may guide the psychiatrist in his choice of procedure in the matter of concluding psychotherapeutic interviews on schedule. This should be done for the sake of both his time and that of his patients, but he should not be unduly dominated by the rule of the clock. Some therapists seem to think that they must terminate interviews on the dot. Prompted by the fear that patients may otherwise take advantage of their indulgence, they will disregard breaking into these patients' communications of highly emotionally charged experiences or interrupting them in the middle of a sentence. I have elaborated upon this erroneous concept in the discussion of the doctor's role in the psychotherapeutic process. I have also warned against having an interview end on a note of more anxiety than can be handled by some patients during the intervals. In general, the suggestion is valid that the routine procedure of concluding an interview should not be charged with an undue amount of overconsideration. The psychiatrist should safeguard against this, since the more routinely this necessary procedure is effected, the less difficult it is for the average patient. This does not exclude consideration for a patient who has done trying psychotherapeutic work or who has recalled upsetting experiences. He should be given sufficient time to collect himself before being required to leave the office, if his need for it is evidenced. The psychiatrist should show the patient further consideration by refraining from immediately pursuing any type of new activity in his presence.

Some patients feel the need to conclude the therapeutic interview themselves before the psychiatrist proceeds to do so. They may do this, at the end of some interviews, either to evade the pursuit of hard therapeutic scrutiny which is under way or to avoid the production of anxiety-arousing, embarrassing, or painful material which is on the patient's mind and on the tip of his tongue.

Other patients feel that they must routinely be the ones to terminate the interviews. Either these patients feel threatened by the impending dependence on a person to whom they would grant the power of deciding when to dismiss them for the day; or they conclude the hour in an attempt to ward off their longing for dependence, which seems fraught with danger for some biographically determined reason; or they conclude the interview because of a need to live up to what appears to them the valid proof of independence, upon which they rely for their alleged security and integrity, and this is their reason for trying to be their own masters.

Motivations of any kind that manifest themselves in these "acting-out" processes, of course, are a reflection of a general interpersonal problem of the patient, just as is any other emotional experience connected with the patient's relationship with the doctor and with any phase of the therapeutic situation. Therefore, the therapist should refrain from responding to these phenomena by either nonverbalized reaction, comment, or therapeutic approach upon their first manifestation. They should be investigated, interpreted, and treated as such, not hastily or inopportunely but in therapeutic congruence with the state of the doctor-patient relationship. The doctor should not approach them until he knows that the patients themselves will not open the discussion of the subject matter. Undesirable self-consciousness and/or unconstructive resistance may be aroused by a premature approach to this type of acting out. Needless to add, in the long run it is not desirable that the patient handle the termination of the interview, because his preoccupation with the clock may easily interfere with relaxation and freedom of production.

# CHAPTER X

## *Termination of Treatment*

WE NOW approach the final problem in intensive psychotherapy—the discussion of the criteria for the conclusion of the treatment and the technique of its termination. Patient and therapist should be satisfied with the results of their psychotherapeutic collaboration if and when the patient has gained a sufficient degree of lasting insight into his interpersonal operations and their dynamics to enable him, in principle, to handle them adequately. This follows from the previously given definition of mental health as being dependent upon the degree of awareness which a person has obtained in regard to his interpersonal processes. As a consequence, the successfully treated mental patient, as he then knows himself, will be much the same person as he is known to others, as H. S. Sullivan puts it (147). This being so, the evaluation of the patient's personality by both patient and psychiatrist should coincide to a very large degree toward the end of the treatment. Out of this coincidence a mutual consensus may frequently be reached between the patient and the therapist about the pending termination of treatment.

The best measuring rod for patients' having attained sufficient insight into the dynamics of their interpersonal processes for therapeutic purposes will be the successful dissolution of their transference experiences and parataxic distortions regarding people and interpersonal situations. This holds true in general and can be especially well evaluated by the changes in the doctor-patient relationship. The experience of and the expression about this relationship must be freed from the previous need of patients for repeating old patterns, parataxic distortions, and extravagant over- and understatements about the personality of and the relationship with the therapist. Signs of compulsive overdependence or spiteful negations of granting the psychiatrist any influence must also have subsided. Psychiatrist and patients will know when this has taken place: first, when the patients' statements pertaining to the therapist become increasingly true to fact; second, when they envisage as a future accomplishment the patients' ability to place realistic evaluation upon the therapist and their relationship with him. To put it in Ferenczi's language: at the time of the termination of treatment, patients should no longer be concerned with fantasies of active or passive castration of and by the psychiatrist or the significant people of their childhood, whose personalities during treatment were invested in the psychiatrist (32).

If the doctor-patient relationship is freed from its distortions, it means, as was previously demonstrated, that the patients are able to see people and situations in general as they *are* rather than as shadows of their past experiences. I mean by this that they are now capable of visualizing not only the psychiatrist but people and interpersonal situations in general, without the errors in appraisal and evaluation which are the unhappy outcome and concomitants of their previous parataxic distortions.

As a rule, this should include the ability of patients to get along with the significant people of their infancy and childhood without the interference of too marked emotional swings. They should have gained a marked degree of awareness of the causes of their previous overattachment or hatred toward these people. They need not love them, but their awareness should be sufficient to enable them to clarify and channel both psychopathological hatred and love within themselves and in their elders. I make a point of this because there seems to be a misconception in the minds of many psychiatrists that learning to hate one's parents is considered a therapeutic accomplishment per se. Quite in contradistinction to this erroneous concept is the true therapeutic goal of gaining independence from one's previous hateful or loving attachments to one's elders and gaining a nondefiant sense of self-value and independence free and apart from their judgment. Hatred and resentment engendered by Oedipal fantasies or by the actual erroneous and damaging pedagogical attitudes and actions of the parents of one's childhood, more often than not, must be experienced in the course of the treatment while striving for independence. However, the maintenance of this hatred toward the parent of today does not constitute a therapeutic goal. The process of revaluation of the relationship of patients with the therapist and others is accompanied by a resolution of their overdependent need for approval and of the disconcerting influence of disapproval from significant people at large. We may recall in this context that dissolution, or at least diminution, of this dependence is an instrument for resolving, or at least for markedly decreasing, the anxiety of mental patients.

This re-establishment of old relationships along new lines, with the accompanying decrease of anxiety, should prepare patients to handle adequately their current interpersonal processes. Similarly, patients should be prepared to meet the vicissitudes of their future life without anxiety or at least with sufficiently diminished anxiety that they can experience them without recurrence of the neurotic or psychotic responses which originally brought them into treatment.

Freud has expressed it this way: the interpretation and working-through of the conflicts from within, which during treatment were artificially aroused by the transference situation or otherwise, should subsequently enable former patients to cope successfully with future conflicts imposed on them by the inevitable vicissitudes of their actual lives (42).

No one living in this era and culture is expected either to be or to remain consistently free from any inklings of anxiety after the termination of treatment. Life will not be "devoid of risks, conflicts, hence anxiety," as Horney puts it, but former patients should potentially be able, after treatment, to solve their conflicts and to spot and resolve their anxiety without the help of a psychiatrist (85).

This marked lessening of anxiety, then, is another indication that the termination of treatment is well timed. It is well to remember again here, in order to understand the far-reaching implications of this statement, that all mental disorders may be understood as an expression of and a means of warding off an unbearable surplus of anxiety. For this reason, the dissolution of the surplus anxiety of patients must be tantamount to counteracting the rise or perpetuation of mental disorder.

Stating that patients should be free of an overdependent need for approval and from the fear of disapproval of significant environmental figures implies another sign of the successful termination of treatment. It signifies that patients are free from the symptoms, anxieties, and inhibitions which previously interfered with their ability for self-realization, that is, with their ability to recognize and use their talents, skills, and powers to their satisfaction, within the realm of their freely established, realistic set of values. This coincides with Fromm's viewpoint that the former patients should have acquired freedom for growth and maturation into predominantly creative, productive personalities (57).*

It follows from what has been said in general throughout this book and in this chapter about termination of treatment that in ending treatment the psychiatrist does not expect perfection in a patient's ability to get along in life. At no point of the treatment has he presented himself to his patients either as a perfect person or as a perfect therapist, and at no point of the treatment should he convey the expectation to patients that he wants them to be either perfect patients or perfect people. This also holds true for indications pointing to the termination of treatment. Patients are not expected to uncover, interpret, and work through all dissociated and repressed interpersonal experiences of their lives (42). Uncovering, interpreting, and working through previously dissociated material can be discontinued when patients attain sufficient awareness of their interpersonal processes, especially in terms of the clarification of their defense mechanisms, and are therefore ready for independent living. This, of course, should include their ability to safeguard against the danger of recurrence of their symptoms and of those problems in living which are beyond their ability to resolve independently. This viewpoint is in contrast to the older, now relinquished, concept of some of Freud's disciples that an analysis is terminated when all repressed childhood memories are uncovered (100).

The aims of intensive psychotherapy as depicted here are seemingly much less ambitious and much more limited than the goals of psychotherapy and the set of values connected with them which were given in Part I. What appears to be a contradiction resolves itself, however, as we realize that the evaluational goals of psycho-

---

* For other suggestions about indications for the termination of treatment offered by classical psychoanalysts see Refs. 31, 72, 99, and the literature quoted by these authors. For the criteria promoted by Alexander and the Chicago Psychoanalytic Institute see Refs. 5 and 6.

therapy as previously enumerated are signposts for therapist and patients for collaboration in treatment and for the patients' own posttherapeutic endeavors. Patients are not expected to reach all these ultimate psychotherapeutic goals during treatment. However, if they accomplish the aims of treatment as cited in this chapter, it may be presupposed that the road is open for the possible eventual posttherapeutic fulfilment of the all-comprehensive goals of treatment which were outlined earlier.

Growth, maturation, and the expansion of personality in the direction of the capability of self-realization, the giving and accepting of love, and forming durable relationships of intimacy are all continuous experiences in living. Their perpetuation and renewal should be an ever present goal throughout the lives of all former patients. After the termination of treatment they should be able to reach out through their own endeavors for the accomplishment of these goals. This was what Freud referred to when he said that psychoanalysis and the therapeutic method aiming at the facilitation of growth and maturation in the human are "interminable" in essence as long as the patient lives and as long as changing mental processes and fluctuating emotional experiences are at work within him and his environment. This does not mean to say, however, that the process of psychoanalytic psychotherapy—that is, of working toward one's change, growth, and maturation with the help of a psychiatrist—is "interminable." This part of a patient's change and recovery through growing insight can fortunately be brought to a "natural end" with many patients (42).

One criterion for tentatively appraising the success of treatment is brought about by the discontinuation of the patient's previous complaints and symptomatology. Another means of evaluation may be given by the patients' sense of regained competence and the corroboration of this sense of competence in terms of actual accomplishment. Sometimes a valid clue may come from what a person thinks and expresses while asleep, that is, in conclusive dreams which point in the direction of termination of the psychotherapeutic process. However, neither one of these indications can be used alone as valid criteria unless it is linked with other signs of the patients' recovery and well-being. The most valid criterion, of course, justifying discontinuation of treatment is offered by the signs of successful dissolution of patients' transference experiences and parataxic distortions which were previously discussed. The reviews of therapeutic accomplishments and the attempts at appraising progress which were mentioned in the chapter on the working-through processes (pp. 141–45) furnish another aid in determining the indications for the termination of treatment.

Should it be felt that still further confirmation is required, it may be wise in some instances to set a tentative date upon which treatment is to be discontinued. The intervening span of treatment may be used as a trial period in which both the patient and the psychiatrist may reach a decision about the desirability of definite termination.

Rank and Ferenczi experimented extensively with this device, the implication, however, being that the date set for termination of treatment should act as therapeutic pressure on the patient. They also required that this date not be rescinded. In cases in which reconsideration proved to be inevitable, continuation of psychoanalysis with another psychiatrist was recommended. After some years of experimentation, this technique was relinquished because it did not fulfil the expected therapeutic promise (33).

It may be wise to give some patients a trial period of living without exchange with the therapist, such as may occur, for instance, because of the therapist's or the patients' vacations. Final treatment may follow, in the course of which patients' interim interpersonal experiences can be checked. Problems brought into focus at this time can still be clarified and worked through then to great therapeutic advantage.

In the case of some other patients, termination of treatment may be indicated before its goals are actually attained. These are the patients to whom the psychoanalytic procedure becomes a way of living in its own right, thus preventing them from ever trying to experiment with the actual business of independent living. They may have to be forced away from intensive psychotherapy into facing the adventures of living. With some of them, treatment may be resumed after a prolonged interval of independent living, with its successes and its failures.

Toward the end of treatment there may be a reappearance of the symptoms which initially brought a patient into psychoanalysis. Sometimes conclusive states of disturbance may also be evidenced. Most of the time neither of these manifestations should be considered a counterindication for the termination of treatment. They are, rather, expressions of the tendency of the personality for real accomplishment. More often than not, these relapses are determined by a patient's tendencies to bring remaining unclarified emotional material into the open for therapeutic reconsideration and solution before treatment is actually discontinued.

It has been previously stated that the decision to discontinue treatment can frequently be reached on the basis of a patient's successful, realistic agreement with the therapist that termination is indicated. Needless to say, there are some patients who may never reach an agreement with the therapist's suggestion that their treatment is nearing the point of termination. A person who has spent a substantial period of time facing his problems with the help of another (the therapist) may be fearful and anxious when faced with the eventuality of giving up that person's collaborative help. Termination of treatment implies exchanging allegiance with a helpful, benevolent guide for a lonely struggle with life strictly on one's own. The tendency of these patients to prolong unduly the psychotherapeutic interrelationship should not call forth either derision or expressions of blame or discouragement from the therapist. He may counteract this reluctance to terminate treatment by fostering the patients' tendencies toward growth and maturation and so encourage them. As we have emphasized throughout this book, every personality harbors such tendencies, no matter how much other parts of the person may at times interfere with their emergence.

Of course, there are some persons whose expectancy from life has become so impoverished and to whom life therefore has so little to offer that they have relinquished all interest in using psychiatric help to realize their remaining assets.

In all other cases this motivation toward health and the ever present potential competence immanent in human beings gives the psychiatrist his chance to be helpful if he is ever mindful of these two great assets. No principles of intensive psychotherapy would have any workable value were these two assets not present in the patient. Neither will these principles of intensive psychotherapy work if the psychiatrist does not address himself simply and with sincerity to the collaborative tendencies of the patient toward the improvement and cure of his emotional difficulties in living.

# PART III
## ADJUNCTS TO INTENSIVE PSYCHOTHERAPY

# CHAPTER XI

## The Attitude of the Psychiatrist toward Intercurrent Events in the Lives of the Patient and of the Therapist

THE dynamics of the psychotherapeutic process have been dealt with from various angles in the writings of both psychoanalysts and other psychiatrists. However, the contents of this chapter have not been the subject of more than occasional scattered comments in the psychiatric literature. Questions pertinent to the attitude of the psychiatrist toward intercurrent events in the patient's life and in his own have been asked repeatedly by younger psychiatrists, and the discussion of these problems is frequently required in the staff conferences of psychoanalytic hospitals. With these considerations in mind I thought it desirable to take them up in a special chapter.

First, I wish to discuss the attitude of the psychiatrist toward special intercurrent events in patients' lives as they may occur outside the treatment situation. Such circumstances would include suicidal attempts, death and bereavement, pregnancy, childbirth, engagement, marriage, divorce, severe illness, accidents, etc. Also included in this category are other emergencies among friends or members of the family, any other significant events in the lives of patients or of those close to them, and important decisions in the patients' own lives. Similarly, I will discuss problems which may arise during the course of treatment regarding significant events in the psychiatrist's own life which inevitably will become known to the patient. Here I refer to such events as illness or death among people close to the therapist, impairment of the doctor's own health, and other significant events in the life of the psychiatrist, his relatives, or his friends.

## 1. SUICIDAL ATTEMPTS

Any patient who has made a suicidal attempt must be approached by the psychiatrist as a person who has felt unhappy, incapacitated, discouraged, or desperate enough to actually try to end his life. A thorough investigation of the validity of the causes for the patient's discouragement, unhappiness, or despair must be the starting point of every therapeutic approach to suicide, or suicidal attempts and fantasies. Careful therapeutic scrutiny should include both the reasons which are in awareness and those which are not. There is a fallacy frequently found not only among lay people but among psychiatrists as well that an unsuccessful suicidal attempt is indicative of the fact that the person was not serious in his suicidal intention. The tendency toward life is powerful enough in every living creature to offset the wish to die. It is this strong motivation to live which is the factor at work in most unsuccessful suicides. The number of patients who stage a suicidal attempt to attract attention is negligibly small. But anyone so lacking in self-respect, so unhappy, lonely, or mentally disordered, that he despairs of getting attention by means other than attempted suicide must be equally in need of psychotherapeutic help.

Many suicidal attempts, especially those of manic-depressives in depressed states, not only are intended to be self-destructive but are also dictated by hostile impulses against significant people in the patient's life or parataxically against the psychiatrist. These hostile impulses are frequently within the patient's awareness, as in the case of the depressed patient who said to his psychiatrist that he would have liked to kill himself if only he could have been sure that it would matter to the doctor. There are patients who are unaware of their destructive tendencies against others which co-determine their suicidal attempts. In these cases part of the treatment, of course, must be to bring into awareness these destructive elements entering into the suicidal attempt. In both cases the causes of the hostile attitude toward others must be therapeutically investigated.

No psychiatrist likes to have his patients try to commit suicide. He may dislike being the recipient of the hostility implied, and he may resent the negative reflections upon his prestige. Of course, this does not imply that concern for the patient's welfare does not play an integral part in the psychiatrist's discomfort in the face of a suicidal attempt. Since an exclusive concern for the patient's welfare conforms with the wishful concept of their role as therapists, many psychiatrists may not be aware of the resentment which, unfortunately, may be aroused in them in their own behalf, by suicidal attempts of their patients. I believe this to be the cause of the error frequently made in starting the psychotherapeutic discussion of a patient's suicidal attempt by taking up the hostile elements entering into it rather than by first inquiring about the elements of unhappiness or despair which prompted it. Careful investigation of the doctor's own reaction is therefore recommended prior to his entering into psychotherapeutic endeavors to clarify the factors motivating the attempted suicide of his patient.

Many patients sense the doctor's discomfort in the face of their suicidal impulses and fantasies. They may try to make use of this knowledge in the service of their resistance and as a means of expressing negative aspects in the doctor-patient relationship. They may try to frighten the doctor, and they may try to use his fright as a way of delaying constructive psychotherapeutic collaboration. In response to this, the therapist should bear in mind that he certainly wishes to help the patient to overcome his suicidal impulses and to prevent them from being carried out. But no psychiatrist can carry the total burden of the responsibility for the self-induced death of his patients. This holds true especially with regard to the unpredictable suicidal impulses of some schizophrenics. The sooner the psychiatrist realizes this, the better for him and his patients. The sooner he imparts this knowledge to the patient, the quicker the bugaboo of threatened suicide will be eliminated as a disturbing factor in the doctor-patient relationship.

Sometimes it may be wise for the therapist to warn the patient against giving in to suicidal impulses while undergoing psychotherapy, since these impulses originate from his present state of mind, and the treatment he is undergoing, i.e., psychotherapy, is a procedure which is aimed at change. In this context the patient might be reminded of the fact that death is irrevocable. Of course, the psychiatrist should not present himself in the omnipotent role of one who is in a position to decide, either in the present or in the future, about the life or death of the patient. He may, however, ardently demonstrate the futility of the patient's undertaking psychotherapy with the reservation of an escape into suicide as an ever present recourse.

As to suicidal preoccupations and fantasies, the word of the German philosopher, Nietzsche, may prove to be helpful while coping with them psychotherapeutically: "The thought of suicide has saved many lives." That is, the knowledge that man is free to end his life if and when its burden becomes unbearable has helped many people to cope with their emotional difficulties in living. In this connection may be mentioned the megalomanic fantasy of some patients who toy with the idea of killing themselves because they wish to remove the decision of time, place, and cause of their death from a power greater than themselves. The psychiatrist should deal with this fantasy in the same way in which he deals with other delusions of grandeur.*

## 2. DEATH OF CLOSE RELATIVES OR FRIENDS

The death of a close relative or friend of the patient is an occasion upon which the psychiatrist may relinquish his professional attitude momentarily. He may wish to offer a personal expression of sympathy or condolence to the patient, if it is called for. Before doing so, however, the therapist must either be sure or make sure that the death is an actual loss to the patient and thus a cause for his bereavement. The deceased may be a person whose death is welcome to the patient because of hatred for him, because of his being a rival of the patient in his relatedness to some other person, or in some other situation. Also his death may be welcomed because he impaired the patient's freedom of action, as might be the case with an elderly invalid who could not be left alone and so was constantly in need of personal care. It is obvious that the psychiatrist is the one person who can least afford to be among those who, because of their own unresolved guilt feelings, adhere to the conventionality of observing rituals of mourning or sympathizing re-

---

* It is not the author's intention in this chapter to deal with the psychopathology of suicide and suicidal attempts per se, but only with those aspects relevant to the attitude of the psychiatrist toward suicidal patients. For information about the psychology and the psychopathology of suicide see Refs. 105, 121, 147, 172, 173, 174, 175.

gardless of whether such expressions are called for in a specific case of death.

On the other hand, a psychiatrist is expected to realize that the death of a hated person may still mean a great loss to a patient, first, because an interpersonal integration may be an asset in an otherwise isolated or lonely person's life, even if it is a hostile one. Second, feelings of hatred regarding certain aspects of the personality of the deceased do not necessarily exclude the simultaneous existence of friendly, tender, and warm tendencies in the mind of the patient toward other more acceptable aspects of the same personality. It could be that, because of the existence of the latter, the death of the otherwise hated person might arouse grief and a sense of loss.

The psychiatrist should also realize that in the case of a lonely patient the death of an invalid on whom he has lavished love and attention and from whom he has received some evidence of acceptance and recognition might cause bereavement and a sense of loss. Some patients may not want to admit this or may even bar it from awareness because of a sense of shame and embarrassment about their loneliness and about the inferior nature of their substituted satisfactions. Of course, all these possible aspects of the patient's relationship with the deceased should be subject to therapeutic scrutiny. This would also apply to the guilt feelings which occur concomitantly with all cases of death within the close environment of a patient. During the process of psychotherapy with a patient who has lost someone close to him, the psychiatrist should bear in mind that the period of mourning will, without psychiatric help, normally free a bereaved person in due time from the maintenance of tie-ups with the deceased.*

Sometimes one sees patients who have lost a beloved one prior to beginning intensive psychotherapy and who, for one reason or another, were deprived, or deprived themselves, of the privilege of mourning the deceased at the time of the loss. The retroactively oriented, paralyzing way of living from which these patients frequently suffer can be favorably influenced if the psychiatrist encourages their indulgence in a period of verbalized belated mourning, especially during the psychotherapeutic interviews.

* For further information see Refs. 2, 44, and 147, p. 50.

If the psychiatrist is not certain from his previous work with the patient about the significance in the patient's life of the death of the friend or relative, he may feel free to say so and to suggest psychotherapeutic investigation, rather than express any personal sympathy before he knows whether or not it is called for in a sense other than a conventional one. A legitimate personal expression of condolence on the part of the therapist is justified and advisable, but mere conventionalities have no place in the relationship between a therapist and his patient.

## 3. PREGNANCY AND CHILDBIRTH

Pregnancy, delivery, and childbirth constitute another group of events in the life of the patient which may call for a temporary nonprofessional response on the part of the psychiatrist. The psychiatrist may express his pleasure at the happiness of the patient upon hearing about her pregnancy or the pending fatherhood of a male patient. He may also inquire about the date of the baby's expected arrival and about the well-being of the expectant mother.

Should the child not be wanted, the psychiatrist should not lose track of the fact that pregnancy remains the great and significant experience of natural productivity and one of physical lust and pleasure to his female patient, regardless of her rejection of motherhood (20, 75). This knowledge has been corroborated by the analysis of the depressions which so many women undergo after voluntary abortions and by the analysis of the depressions and other mental disorders which are observed in women who do not have children for one reason or another.

Mothers frequently accept a child warmly upon its arrival, although it was unwanted while carried, if they are not seriously disturbed and if their relationship with the significant people of their past and present life is predominantly a benign one. It is well for the psychiatrist to keep this in mind while conducting the psychoanalytic course of treatment with the future mother.

In the case of psychotherapy with the father, the psychiatrist should not overlook the fact that, to most men, their wife's pregnancy is a welcome sign of their virility, irrespective of their actual wish to procreate.

The parents' predilection regarding the sex of the newcomer must be listened to with the possibility in mind of its being determined within or outside the patient's awareness, either by the wish or by the repugnance of the thought that the newcomer may be a replica of the respective parent himself or of his or her partner. Consideration or refutation of the expectations of other members of the family may also enter the picture within or outside the patients' awareness. Conformance with all types of conventionalities frequently colors the attitude of the prospective parents toward their baby, regardless of the actual significance of these conventionalities for the lives, tastes, and decisions of the prospective parents themselves. Once the psychiatrist has evidenced his personal understanding of the significance of this important event in his patient's life, psychoanalytic scrutiny of all its emotional implications should be encouraged. Technique and method, of course, are the same as in psychotherapeutic work regarding any other event of a similarly intense emotional significance in the life of the patient.

There has been some discussion about the question of whether or not a pregnant woman should discontinue her analysis, lest painful or anxiety-arousing material might be stirred up and interfere with a smooth-running pregnancy. In my opinion it is preferable, *as a rule*, to clarify potentially disturbing emotional factors in the life of a pregnant woman rather than to leave this material undiscussed and free to influence a patient one way or another outside her knowledge and, therefore, outside her control. Clarification may be for the benefit of the expectant mother as well as for the benefit of the child which she carries. It has been my experience that intensive psychotherapy during pregnancy will not undesirably influence the course of the pregnancy if the therapist has been successful in conveying the afore-mentioned attitude to the patient: that pregnancy as such is, in principle, a positive experience in a woman's life, regardless of its possible negative aspects under special conditions. Delivery may be approached in a similar vein.

If a former patient's pregnancy and delivery are forthcoming as events which played an integral part in a preceding analysis of some duration, the psychoanalyst may even go to see the parents and the newcomer, if such a step can be made by him as a matter of course.

Except for seriously disordered patients who were markedly

mixed up about their sex role, I have not found any confirmation of Freud's conception that women experience childbirth as equivalent to at last coming into possession of a penis of their own. Perhaps Freud himself realized later that this conception was among those which called for a revision, when he stated in his *New Introductory Lectures* that he had lived to see that he had not obtained reliable knowledge about female psychosexuality (46).

What I did find, in concurrence with other authors, was that the more or less happy expectation of a baby is co-determined not only by the emotional aspects of the mother's relationship with the father but also frequently and more specifically by the enjoyment she gets in intercourse with the father of the baby.

Great attention should be paid to the relationship of the expectant mother with her own mother. This is another component which colors the emotional factors entering into pregnancy and delivery, frequently outside the patient's awareness. The importance of this factor cannot be overestimated. I have seen patients abort without any physical reason. Their psychoanalytic work uncovered the fact that it was because motherhood seemed unbearable, owing to the unrecognized intense hatred of the pregnant patient toward her own mother. These patients felt that they could not give birth to a child either because that would make them similar to the hated mothers or for fear that their children might hate them as they hated their mothers.

There is another factor which should not be neglected in a psychotherapeutic consideration of childbirth. This is the element of sexual gratification entailed in the mother's delivery of the baby. This is apt to be kept a secret from others by most women, if not barred from their own awareness. In this culture most women prefer to stress the pain of labor only, if for no other reason than in order to impress their husbands. They play up the fact that menstruation, pregnancy, and childbirth are the only experience of one sex which cannot be experienced by the other. It is true, of course, that erection and ejaculation, as such, cannot be experienced by the female either; but the concomitant orgastic sensations are an experience which both sexes have in common. In this connection I would like to mention a side issue, which I believe to be worth the attention of the psychiatrist. Pregnancy and delivery, as experiences of genuine natural productivity and satisfaction, are legitimately charged with an appreciable amount of emotional and physical importance. If so, is it as desirable as the modern American obstetrician claims to anesthetize women routinely during delivery? Or could it be that the price these women pay for being protected from the pains of labor is too high, since at the same time it deprives them of experiencing in full awareness the culminating act of their creativeness (127)? I believe that psychiatric investigation of the possible psychopathological consequences of this emotional deprivation is indicated. I have encouraged several pregnant patients to ask their obstetricians to refrain from anesthetizing them at least during the final act of delivery, if their confinement was normal. The patients were grateful for the experience to which they submitted themselves in following this suggestion. For obvious reasons the same cannot be said about most of their obstetricians. Recently, some psychoanalytically trained obstetricians had encouraging success in eliminating anesthetics while delivering women who were adequately trained and enlightened previous to and during childbirth (101).

A thorough investigation of all the emotional factors inside and outside awareness which can be uncovered in men and women regarding pregnancy and childbirth is recommended, of course, in connection with each expectant patient's psychoanalytical treatment.

The influence exerted by pregnancy, childbirth, and lactation on the baby's older siblings and on their interrelationships with the expectant, the birth-giving, and the nursing mother is another psychoanalytically important aspect of these events.

The method and technique employed in this part of intensive psychotherapy do not differ, of course, from the therapeutic principles discussed throughout this book.

## 4. ENGAGEMENT, MARRIAGE, AND DIVORCE

The decision for engagement, marriage, or divorce or any such crucial steps in a patient's life should be discouraged by the psychiatrist while the patient is under intensive psychotherapy. The goal of psychotherapy is a change in the patient's personality Neither he nor the psychiatrist can know ahead of time what the result of this change will be. It is to be assumed, therefore, that the patient is in no position to know whether commitments made prior to this change may prove desirable in the future. In some cases this is so obvious that the psychiatrist is justified in demanding outright that such decisions be postponed. He may even go so far, at times, as to deem it advisable that treatment be discontinued if the patient does not follow his suggestion. The postponement of all vital decisions until treatment has been terminated is one of the basic rules in classical psychoanalysis.

On the other hand, there may be interpersonal conditions involved in a patient's problems of engagement, marriage, or divorce about which immediate steps should be taken because their hanging in mid-air interferes with, or even blocks, the patient's efforts to learn how to live, his progress, and his further treatment. This may be true especially in difficult premarital or marital situations which existed prior to a patient's entering treatment or which were even instrumental in his decision to seek psychiatric help.

This suggestion of two opposite alternatives implies that it takes all the wisdom and perspicacity of the psychiatrist to decide in which of the two directions to go with an individual patient, depending on the multitude of intangible intricacies which determine the specific life and treatment situation of each patient in question. Needless to say, the psychiatrist should never have a patient make such a decision before having listened intently to the patient's story. Any decision must also be preceded by the patient's and the doctor's extensive collaborative endeavor to investigate, evaluate, and interpret all the available pertinent data. These should include the scrutiny of conscious and unconscious motivations operating in his own life and, in the presence of adequate data, a tentative appraisal of the personality and of the motivations of his partner.

Some patients evade the issue of investigating the validity of the motivations and reasons for their decisions by acting upon them during intervals between psychoanalytic sessions. Serious attention should be paid to the actual and to the parataxic elements determining such behavior. It should be subjected to thorough scrutiny, as to its various possible aspects, each of which may give further important clues to the understanding of the dynamics of a patient's personality and disorder. Some aspects of a patient's hasty act may be its futility, its character of resistance or of adolescent rebellion. And, last but not least, it may be due to fear of the psychiatrist's interference with a decision the validity of which the patient himself is usually doubtful about if he feels compelled to rush into it indiscreetly.

These foregoing examples are only a few from a much larger group of possible motivations, evidencing themselves in types of therapeutically undesirable attitudes toward crucial decisions, which the therapist may encounter in his patients. He may feel annoyed and irritated by such attitudes. If so, he must make sure about the exact nature of his irritation. Is its rise in response to patients' disregard of what is known to be a valid psychotherapeutic principle? Or is it because the contents of their premature and hastily made decisions are in contrast to the beneficial resolution which the therapist wished to see chosen by the patient? The first reaction is in keeping with his mandate as psychiatrist; the latter, however, would be out of step with his role. It would be the "countertransference" reaction of a "father-or-mother-knows-better" variety of psychiatrist.

There are some patients who feel called upon to make important marital decisions shortly before they begin their psychoanalytic treatment. These are generally people who by their pre-analytic acting-out processes wish to prove something which is not true, both to themselves and to their future psychiatrist. They are motivated by their reluctance to face the anxiety engendered not only by their own awareness of their interpersonal difficulties but more so by sharing this knowledge with someone else. In this connection I remember a patient who married hastily two months prior to beginning treatment. Having heard, as she put it, that the psychoanalytic process might entail the discovery and discussion of a person's homosexual problems, she wanted to begin her treatment with the record of a satisfactory heterosexual adjustment.

This undesirable form of acting out her resistance against and her fear of the potential discoveries about herself turned out to be instrumental in unnecessarily prolonging the duration of her treatment.

## 5. REQUESTS FOR ADVICE

The next point for discussion is the problem of other crucial decisions in the intercurrent life of a patient and the attitude of the therapist toward the patients' requests for advice. Many patients will try to get the advice of the psychiatrist about how to proceed when doubtful about a decision, be it a crucial one of the variety mentioned in the preceding chapter or a minor decision in everyday life. As previously mentioned in the discussion of the role of the therapist, his job is to give advice and guidance regarding the course of the therapeutic procedure. He also advises patients about the means to be used for gaining awareness of the elements in their developmental history and in their present life-circumstances which enter into his decision.

Every now and then the psychiatrist may also be called upon actively to help the patient decide about life-arrangements to facilitate or impede the psychotherapeutic process. Will it expedite psychotherapy if the patient lives in his parents' home, in a hospital, nursing-home, or boarding-house, while undergoing psychoanalytic psychotherapy? Should he take a job, half-time or full-time, continue college attendance, etc.? These are questions about which the therapist may be justified in acting in a direct, practical, advisory capacity. In all other cases of practical decisions, the patient should be encouraged to be his own adviser. Psychoanalytic investigation will acquaint him with the personality elements pertinent to his decision, and either of two outcomes should be counted upon. The patient should either be able to make up his own mind, based on his new insight, or he should be encouraged to postpone his decision until a time when he will be capable of making a decision on his own. In this context psychiatrists should recall what has been conveyed throughout the preceding chapters: psychotherapy is a process aimed at the growth and ultimate matureness of the patient. Giving practical advice to patients keeps them in the state of immature dependence upon the judgment and guidance of others, in which they lived as children with regard to their parents and teachers. The dynamics of the psychotherapeutic process imply that the patient at times puts the psychiatrist parataxically in the role of authoritative figures of his previous life.

As we have seen, therapeutic investigation of what the patient is living through in these transference experiences furthers his breaking away from the patterns of his previous dependent adherence to authority outside himself. If the therapist offers encouragement to patients' parataxic expectations by actually falling into the role of practical adviser, he retards the process of insight into the immature character of such expectations; hence he retards the process of resolving them.

Let me repeat from the standpoint of the patient what was previously discussed from the viewpoint of the doctor. In the long run, the patient appreciates it if the psychiatrist does not comply with his request for direct practical advice, no matter how much he may be pressing the doctor for it at the time. His innate tendency toward health, growth, and maturation will eventually be greater than his time-bound wish for the type of help and advice that may interfere with his motivation toward health and independence.

## 6. SEVERE ILLNESS AND ACCIDENTS

The next group of intercurrent events which must be discussed in this context comprises severe illness and accidents. If a patient suffers a severe physical illness or has an accident while under psychiatric treatment, the psychiatrist should feel free to make his concern and sympathy evident to the patient.

The nature of the illness or the accident may be such that it does not preclude therapeutic discussions. If this is so, it may frequently be well for the psychiatrist to go to see the patient professionally every now and then as long as the patient cannot come to see him. This is especially recommended in cases in which the illness or accident entails serious emotional problems of some variety for the patient. It may mean the loss of a limb in an accident. The loss of an income-producing job may be due to illness. There may be impairment of appearance by lasting scars or the death-blow of any hope for an impending marriage and healthy progeny because of a chronic infectious disease, etc.

In the face of an illness which has befallen his patient, the psychiatrist, by all means, should not behave like a parlor-variety "psychoanalyst." By that I mean he should be sure not to jump immediately to glib conclusions about the "unconscious reasons" or about the "psychosomatic aspects" or the "secondary gain of illness," as motivating the onset of the sickness or the occurrence of the accident. Unfortunately, these not infrequent reactions on the part of psychiatrists may seriously interfere with the ultimate physical and emotional recovery of the patient.

All diseases and many accidents have their emotional aspects, in addition to the physical and material ones. All patients must be given time to recover from the immediate results of the shocking experience of the realization of their impairment. The average patient who has been indoctrinated in psychoanalytic thinking will reach the point of pondering to himself and of talking to his therapist on his own volition about the psychiatric aspects of his predicament. For obvious reasons this will happen more quickly, as a rule, the less the psychiatrist presses the patient. An example in point which came to my attention recently is that of a patient who had an accident while driving his car. This man was an excellent driver who did not remember having had an accident during the twenty years since he had obtained his driver's license. While under treatment, he backed into another car one day while parking, with the result that he seriously damaged his own car. His spontaneous comments during the psychoanalytic interview the following day were to the effect that the accident had frightened him in a very specific way. He said it was so unlike him to have such a thing happen that he suspected that inattention to what he was doing had caused the accident. Intense preoccupation with some severe interpersonal problems, the nature of which were unknown to him, appeared to have absorbed his attention. He decided upon his own volition to drive back to the place of the accident, as soon as the repair-shop returned his car. He hoped that being confronted with the place again might help him discover the contents of the preoccupations which had so disastrously interfered with the concentration of his attention on his driving.

While conducting the psychotherapeutic discussion of the emotional aspects of a physical illness with a patient, the psychiatrist should bear in mind that the function of the illness need not at all be merely a negative one. Temporary physical illness has a constructive role in the course of the lives of many people, whether they are mental patients or virtually healthy people. I will not elaborate further on this topic. The philosophy of illness has been discussed by the great medical men of all times and nationalities (164, 165, 167).

Psychoanalytic psychiatrists, in their eagerness to discover the immediate specific meaning of a patient's physical symptomatology, may have been in danger of losing track of the broader philosophical aspects of physical disease. Research has been directed toward the discovery of the frequently nonconstructive meaning of the start of a physical ailment in a specific setting. This should always be done on the basis of respect for and acceptance of the possibility that there also may be constructive philosophical aspects at the root of a physical ailment and in the background of its onset at a given time.

I am afraid that the unprejudiced attitude of the psychiatrist toward these problems may sometimes be impaired by various facts. The physical illness of a mental patient who cannot keep his psychotherapeutic appointments entails an unwelcome temporary reduction of the psychiatrist's income. Going to see the patient causes an equally unwelcome interference with the smooth running of his hour-by-hour schedule. It may prove helpful to the psychiatrist to be aware of these humanly understandable, but nonetheless unacceptable, trends in his attitude toward the patient. It may help him to safeguard against their interfering with a therapeutically constructive attitude toward intercurrent physical illnesses and accidents in the lives of his patients.

In concluding the discussion of intercurrent events during the course of patients' treatment, I shall now take up the discussion of significant events in the life of the psychiatrist.

## 7. SIGNIFICANT EVENTS IN THE LIFE OF THE PSYCHIATRIST

Inevitably, in the course of a long analysis there may be times when a psychiatrist feels below par physically or emotionally during a psychotherapeutic interview. As long as he feels that his condition does not interfere with his work with the patient, there is no reason to mention it, since it may merely offer a distraction to the patient or, even worse, burden him needlessly. However, should the patient notice something, it is recommended that the issue not be evaded. Without being unnecessarily self-conscious, the psychiatrist may offer a simple direct statement of facts, with the additional comment that, to the best of his knowledge and judgment, his present condition is not likely to interfere with his work with the patient. If he or the patient feels that there is marked interference, it is preferable to say so frankly. There is then the alternative of either trying to continue the interview despite the handicap or to discontinue that specific interview. The frank admission that the psychiatrist is human and not infallible shows far more respect and consideration for the patient than evasion would. It may also contribute to the process of maturing, which is part of the goal of the psychotherapeutic process.

It is, of course, possible for a significant occurrence, such as death, marriage, childbirth, or divorce, to take place in the life of the psychiatrist while a patient is under treatment. It may then be advisable for the psychiatrist to interrupt treatment for a sufficiently long period of time to take care of his preoccupation with his own affairs. As treatment is resumed, he may unassumingly comment upon his reasons for the interruption and add that he is now ready for work. He should bear in mind that the patient may wish to express condolences, congratulations, or merely make a comment, and so he should not fail to give him an opening to do so.

In this connection, I recall a disturbed schizophrenic who had heard of the death of a very close friend of the psychiatrist. The patient was completely blocked in his communication when the psychiatrist first resumed work with him following the death of the friend until the psychiatrist made a remark to the effect that she realized he knew of her loss.

On the other hand, I recall the example of a psychiatrist who was engaged to be married. Several of her young women patients who happened to have heard about the engagement expressed skepticism as to the psychiatrist's ability to concentrate upon her work with them. She replied that, had she doubted her ability to do so, she would temporarily have discontinued seeing patients. Following this, psychotherapeutic work was resumed as usual.

It has been advocated that patients be given credit for the possible discernment of intercurrent instances of physical or emotional involvements in the life of the psychiatrist. It should also be kept in mind, however, that patients are people absorbed in their own troubles who are trained to look upon the psychiatrist as a participant observer of their difficulties. The attention given by the patient to the life and the problems of the psychiatrist should therefore not be overestimated, either.

These suggestions may suffice to facilitate the psychiatrist's orientation to the problem of his attitude to patients with regard to intercurrent events in his life.

# CHAPTER XII

## Contacts with Relatives

DURING the years when only neurotics were accepted for psychoanalytic treatment, there was a prevalent rule against the psychiatrist's seeing the relatives of the patient if it possibly could be avoided. The concept behind this was that, in the long run, the patient himself would produce the data, which one might try to gather more quickly as collateral information from relatives. There was another aspect relevant to the therapist's not seeing the significant people of the patient's environment: since they were instrumental in the rise of the patient's disturbances, their being seen by the therapist might deprive the patient of the therapeutically valid security of having found someone who would side with him, if necessary, against the powerful and conflict-provoking environmental figures. It was also assumed that it would be easier for the psychiatrist to form his own judgment about questions of interrelatedness between the patient and his environment from the changing pertinent data which the patient would produce in the course of treatment than from some immediate contact with the relatives.

Many psychiatrists still feel that way. I personally, and many of my psychiatric friends also, like to see a significant person of the patient's environment, depending on the patient's agreement. I believe that collateral information, if used with discretion, may speed the total course of treatment. I also think it is helpful for the psychiatrist to gather an impression of his own about the significant people in the patient's life, to whom the patient himself will refer time and again with changing evaluational references. Last but not least, there may be some patients to whose relatives the psychiatrist may wish to transmit enlightening and educational information about the nature of the patient's disorder and its interpersonal implications. Of course, careful attention must be given to the timing of interviews with relatives in connection with the state of the treatment and of the patient's relationship with the therapist.

Collateral information from relatives will help to speed the psychotherapeutic process and not obstruct it only if the psychiatrist listens, ever mindful of the potential unreliability of such information. The data may be distorted because the relatives of a neurotic patient are apt to be neurotic themselves, so that their information suffers from misrepresentation, just as does that of the patient. Also, a relative who is aware of his damaging effect upon the patient prior to the start of treatment is likely to change at least the nuance of his information if not more, in an attempt to make his part in the rise of the patient's disorder abstruse. Checking the data of the patient against those of the relatives is one way to counteract the danger of being misled by the unreliability of the relative's information.

Another source of possible misinformation is due to misinterpretation caused by the psychiatrist's errors in appraisal. These errors may be brought about by his positive transference to the patient or his negative attitude toward the relative. Less frequently the source of the error may be the psychiatrist's dependent attitude toward the authority represented by the social or financial status of a relative. The twofold supply of information from patient and relative can be helpful if the psychiatrist is alert to the intrinsic danger involved in gaining data in this way.

Another significant point to which attention should be paid is the question of which relative of a patient is to be seen by the doctor. The type of information given and sought by each member of the family—father, mother, sibling, uncle, cousin, etc.—will vary, depending upon the role of each of these people in the family group and on their relationship to one another and to the patient now and in his premodbid days. Accordingly, each relative's data will have to be evaluated differently.

If a relative expresses the wish to see the psychiatrist, the doctor must first inquire from the patient as to his attitude toward it. If the patient has no objections and if, according to his own judgment, the doctor's seeing the relative does not interfere with the course of the treatment at the time, he may give him an appointment. Under no circumstances should the psychiatrist interview a relative without the patient's knowing it. Even if the psychiatrist is willing to do so at the expense of violating the principle of mutual sincerity governing the doctor-patient relationship, it would still be contraindicated. The psychiatrist cannot depend upon the reliability of the relative to keep their meeting a secret from the patient, nor can he depend fully upon his own ability at all times not to give an inadvertent clue to its having taken place.

If the patient consents to the psychiatrist's seeing a relative and, more so, if he requests him to do so on his own volition, the patient's motives in doing so should be investigated before his consent or request is acted upon. This consent or wish may be fully legitimate. The patient may feel that he can rely upon the judgment of the psychiatrist who asks for permission to interview the relative. Moreover, he may personally consider it advisable for the psychiatrist to meet significant people of his environment and have them submitted to the psychiatrist's own evaluational judgment.

Other patients may be motivated by illegitimate reasons, such as a sense of overdependence on their doctor or by the wish to use the psychiatrist as a good mother versus the relative as the bad mother. Still another group of patients may wish to have the psychiatrist and significant environmental figures of their lives meet, so that the psychiatrist may enlighten and educate the relatives about the patient's problems and needs. Frequently it will prove helpful to recommend or hand to relatives good popular literature explaining the nature of mental disorder and of the psychotherapeutic procedure (12, 34, 93, 96, 97, 116, 117).

In the case of neurotic patients who are not too disturbed, educating relatives should not be the job of the psychiatrist. As the patient matures under the influence of successful treatment, he should, on his own, be able to secure the understanding of the relatives for his problems and needs and, later on, for his specific way of living. In the case of neurotic children and of relatives who are seriously disturbed themselves, this expectation does not hold true.

Psychotic patients may need the help of the psychiatrist in enlightening and handling relatives. Suggestions about the doctor's means of doing this will be offered later.

When the therapist has excluded any illegitimacy of motives

influencing either a patient's consent or his request that the doctor see a relative, he should try to reach a tentative evaluational conclusion about the reasons motivating the relative's request. These reasons may largely determine the reliability and usefulness of the information offered by the relative. It may not always be easy to reach such a conclusion because, more often than not, the relative will try to display a misleading, defensive attitude in an attempt to screen underlying motivations, about which the doctor is not supposed to know.

Does the relative wish to see the psychiatrist in the spirit of collaboration and genuine interest in the welfare of the patient? Is he prompted by the wish to give or to receive pertinent information which may be helpful in gearing his attitude toward the patient? Is his request determined by a wish to meet the doctor who is supposed to help the patient in the family? The latter reason should not be frowned upon as a rule, since it may not be due simply to vague curiosity, with its attendant nuisance value, but may be prompted by an understandable wish to contribute in any way possible to the patient's recovery.

Other relatives may feel the need to see the psychiatrist for reasons of their own, some of them legitimate, some not. For valid reasons, they may wish to see the psychiatrist to gain help in understanding the predicament of the patient and in regard to the interpersonal difficulties which have arisen between the patient and the relative prior to and during the patient's mental disturbance.

Still another group of significant people from the patient's immediate environment, realizing that poor handling of the patient by them could have contributed to the rise of the disorder, may come to unburden themselves and to find relief from their feelings of guilt about the possibility of their traumatic role in the development of the patient's disorder.

Unfortunately, quite a number of relatives are prompted by illegitimate reasons in their request to see the psychiatrist. This may be due to the wish of all too many significant environmental figures not to relinquish a part in the psychotherapeutic process, as well as a hold over the patient. The psychiatrist may expect advice from these people on how to treat the patient, offered with the rationalization that they have known the patient much longer than the psychiatrist has.

Despite these and similar trying situations with relatives, the psychiatrist should do his best to live up to the expectation that he is an expert in handling interpersonal relationships. Mistreatment of relatives may cause unfavorable repercussions in the relative-patient-doctor relationship and, quite likely, will work to the detriment of the patient both at the time and later. I believe it will help the psychiatrist in his endeavor to meet the patient's relative in the right spirit if he will keep the following facts in mind. The relatives are strangers on their first visit to the psychiatrist and therefore, in contrast to the patient under treatment, have not been given the opportunity to develop a relationship of trust and confidence with the psychiatrist such as the patient has developed in the course of his continuous interviews.

Moreover, the relative in his own prejudiced way, which, after all, is the way of the average psychiatrically uneducated citizen, is justified for many reasons in his dislike or hatred for the psychiatrist who is treating a member of the family. An initial reason for these adverse feelings might be that the secret that there is a mental patient in the family has to be given away to the psychiatrist. Another reason might be that the relative, who knows that the mental patient is supposed to tell the psychiatrist whatever occupies his mind, will realize that the doctor is also going to hear about all the "sacred" secrets of the family. Many psychiatrists know from their practice how frequently patients, prior to beginning treatment, have been cautioned against giving away the secrets of the family. A third origin of relatives' dislike of the psychiatrist may well be that among these secrets will be the blunders made by various members of the family in their dealing with the patient, which have contributed to the rise or development of his mental disorder. The fact that psychotherapy may produce changes in the type of integration which the patient has accomplished with various members of the family will also be among the sources of relatives' antagonism toward the psychiatrist. This hostility constitutes a threat to the unprepared relatives because it sometimes calls for concomitant changes in integration on their part.

For instance, a formerly obsessional patient may no longer continue to focus his interest on overtrimness or pedantic correctness in his contacts with things and people. This may make it necessary for the partner, who has been geared to the obsessional ways of the patient, either to make a considerable adjustment in his turn or to run the risk of having the relationship disintegrate.

A patient who was previously markedly submissive may gain inner independence in the course of his treatment, which again either his partner or perhaps a parent may not be prepared to grant him. Hence these significant people in the patient's life would feel that the psychiatrist did them a great disservice.

After working with the psychiatrist, a person who had formerly been aloof and self-engulfed may become more outgoing and more interested in relating himself to others. The familiar interpersonal adjustment of the members of the family to the patient will be thrown into confusion by the change in his personality. The result of this may be resentment against the psychiatrist who had been instrumental in the patient's change.

A previously domineering person may mature in the course of his treatment so that he will be ready for a personal interrelatedness on the level of mutual acceptance. His supposedly submissive partner will be faced with a very difficult problem, irrespective of whether or not he wishes or is able to adjust to this change.

A patient may overcome the symptom of frigidity through psychotherapy. This newly realized sexual aliveness may conceivably release a great amount of anxiety in her husband, who for many years had found it necessary to gear himself to his wife's inhibited ways.

A husband or wife who had shared the other's lack of interest in procreation may develop a wish for children in the course of his or her treatment. Again the partner is faced with the adjustment to a new life-problem for the creation of which he may not thank the psychiatrist.

There are further understandable reasons for the fact that many relatives feel that the psychiatrist who is treating a member of the family is their enemy. From the standpoint of the family, the psychiatrist may frequently side temporarily with the so-called "peculiarities and oddities" of the patient. What is more, the patient may quote the psychiatrist in defense of his own position against the relatives. At this point it will be most propitious for the further course of treatment to have the psychiatrist forthrightly maintain the attitude he has taken. He most assuredly should not be induced by the puzzled or disgruntled member of the family to shift his attitude toward the patient. For instance, such a change could happen under the pressure of anxiety of the perhaps powerful or financially important relative, or in hospitals, under the pressure of anxiety in a younger member of the medical staff regarding the disapproval of the superintendent. The doctor should be mindful of this danger, so that he can safeguard against it if it arises.

Relatives' distrust of the psychiatrist again may be aroused when a patient appears more ill or when his behavior becomes worse, owing to symptoms being temporarily stirred up by psychotherapeutic scrutiny.

A suggestion that may be of value to some psychiatrists is dictated by personal experience. If the doctor feels threatened by a sense of impatience or irritation toward relatives, he should make an attempt to visualize them temporarily as if they were his patients, that is, in the light of the genetics and dynamics of their own interpersonal background. With all these suggestions in mind, the psychiatrist should be able to avoid the sense of despair which Freud professed regarding the presenting problems of disturbed relatives (37).

Prior to seeing a patient's relatives, the psychiatrist should talk over with the patients, from their viewpoint, which of their communications to the doctor they wish him to discuss or not to discuss with the relative. Frequently, the answer may be, "Tell him whatever you want to, provided you tell *me* afterward." If, however, patients do have definite suggestions, the doctor should abide by them. Sometimes joint conferences between relative, patient, and doctor may be indicated and helpful. This may be a means of relieving tension for both relatives and patients regarding further interviews between relatives and doctor. In the case of an inarticulate or disturbed psychotic, the psychiatrist, of course, must use his own judgment.

As a rule, it can be recommended that the relatives be encouraged to do most of the talking. Frequently they are under the influence of tension, preoccupation with their own role, and exhaustion engendered by the conditions which preceded the final decision for the patient to undertake treatment. When relatives ask the psychiatrist for information, the doctor should be able to make many clarifying remarks which will help the relative and the patient and, at the same time, will avoid interference with the patient's legitimate wish for privacy. Relatives who for legitimate reasons are seeking contact with a patient's therapist should never be denied the privilege of seeing the doctor, solely on the basis of safeguarding against the use of the patient's confidential material.

There is no need for discussion of contacts with relatives who are genuinely collaborative, willing, and able to comprehend and go along with the problems and changes which arise from the disturbance of a mental patient. A remark should be added, though, about contacts with those relatives who are or pretend to be overappreciative. The doctor must safeguard against such flattering play on his quest for prestige. Otherwise, he may be tempted to indulge in overoptimistic fantasies, thereby deviating from his professional line of realistic appraisal of the patient's present condition and future progress and of his own therapeutic role.

In the case of disturbed psychotic patients, especially inarticulate ones, collateral information from relatives will frequently prove to be indispensable. The therapist can use this information as a guide during periods of treatment in which no direct information can be secured from the patient. In his contact with relatives of psychotic patients, the therapist must remember that the relatives themselves are frequently disturbed, not infrequently rather defensive, and at times malevolent. This is less frequently true with the relatives of neurotics. If possible, he should try to find one benevolent figure in the entourage of the psychotic patient whom he can interest in the collaboration and handling of the rest of the relatives. The benevolent relative may help the psychiatrist in his efforts to reawaken the patient's interest in testing outer reality and in accepting interpersonal reorientation. He may also be useful in assisting the therapist in his efforts to encourage the patient's reacceptance of himself and in resuming relationships with others.

Some members of Chestnut Lodge Sanitarium have recently been successful in favorably influencing the course of treatment of psychotic patients by teaching the mothers, through personal interviews and letters, how to change their behavior to the patient. Encouraged by the favorable results of this approach in children's mental hygiene centers, various attempts are made to obtain further accomplishments along these lines with adolescent and adult psychotics in many hospitals throughout the country. The patient's therapist either personally sees the relative at regular intervals or secures the help of another psychiatrist for the job of enlightening and training the person. Both doctors keep in constant collaborative contact. Some hospitals are attempting to reach the same goal by conducting group-therapy sessions jointly for young psychotics and their mothers. (Cf. forthcoming paper of Abrahams [Washington, D.C.].)

In speaking about the significance of securing the help of patients' relatives, we would also like to include other figures, who may have been equally important, or even more so, in the early life of the patient, such as nurses, kindergarten teachers, friends of older siblings, etc.

Regarding interviews with a patient's own friends, *mutatis mutandis*, the same suggestions are offered for the contacts with relatives, with this addendum: For obvious reasons, the motivations to protect themselves are less frequent and far less profound in friends and contemporaries of patients than they are in relatives. Therefore, there is less danger of emotional distortion and less interference with the evaluation and representation of their information. More often than not, they may be able to make valid contributions to the general understanding of the patients' environmental history as well as their difficulties in living with their families.

The visits of relatives and friends with hospitalized psychotics have always been a moot problem with institutional therapists. By and large, they have been inclined to eliminate or curtail visits if they seemed to make the patients more disturbed. Generally speaking, this practice seems undesirable to me because it encourages prejudice and makes for weird fantasies regarding mental hospitals. What is of more importance than this, however, is the repeated experience which every hospital therapist has had with the majority of the patients about people coming to see them. The visit of their relatives may disturb and upset them temporarily, and, while discussing an impending visit, they may seriously consider declining to see their relatives. Yet, when the visitor actually arrives, it becomes evident with a great number of patients that they have wanted the visit after all. The sense of belonging, the heightening of their self-respect, and the increased prestige in the eyes of other patients caused by visits from relatives and friends mean so much to the hospitalized psychotic that he should not be deprived of them, although at times patients do react with what appears to be a temporary setback in their progress. Autobiographical publications of previously hospitalized people who have recovered also point in the direction of the desirability of patients' receiving visitors (4, 8, 15).

Sometimes visits of significant people, if rightly timed, may turn out to be even more than an immediate psychotherapeutic adjuvant, as in the following examples: A young schizophrenic girl harbored the memory of a beloved nursemaid who had meant more to her than anyone else throughout her life and allegedly still did. The nursemaid came to visit the patient in the hospital. This gave the patient an opportunity to revaluate the significance of this relationship for the reality of her present age level. This marked the beginning of a definite improvement in the patient's environmental orientation and general condition.

Another young schizophrenic considered her governess to be her only real friend during her childhood days and thereafter. During her late teens she had consummated a homosexual relationship with this governess. This significant figure was invited to visit the patient while she was still sufficiently disturbed to need hospitalization. Her previous teen-age crush and her homosexual tie subsided and were replaced by a noncommittal friendly relationship with full appreciation of the present assets and liabilities of the beloved childhood figure. Again this reorientation became the starting point for a definite move toward improvement and progress.

There are patients, of course, for whom visits are inadvisable, either because of a relative's inability to approach the patient adequately or because of the reluctance of the patient to see him. In such instances the staff members of psychiatric hospitals should encourage the patients' relatives to visit the hospital even if the patient cannot see them. The relatives should be encouraged to see the superintendent, the therapist, and/or a nurse, as the case may be. That way prejudice and ill feeling may be counteracted and an opportunity be given for the possible exchange of valuable information which may ultimately accrue to the patient's benefit.

In the last analysis, the previous statements about therapeutic contacts with patients may be applied, *mutatis mutandis*, to relatives as well. The psychotherapist will be capable of handling these contacts successfully to the extent to which he attempts to address himself to his patients' relatives, more mindful of their potential assets than of their actual liabilities. It is a psychiatrist's privilege to bring to the fore the assets of the people who contact him professionally.

# REFERENCE LIST

# REFERENCE LIST

This reference list cannot and is not intended to form a complete list of the publications pertaining to the subject matters discussed in this book. From the host of pertinent writings, those were selected which were most helpful to the author in increasing her own knowledge throughout the years and in the preparation of this text. The choice was also determined by the consideration of the specific representative value of a publication in its own field and by its value as a source of over-all information.

1. ABRAHAM, KARL. A Revised Psychopathology, Internat. J. Psycho-Analysis, pp. 271 ff., 1941.
2. ———. A Short Study of the Development of the Libido Viewed in the Light of Mental Disorders. In: Selected Papers, pp. 418–76. London: Hogarth Press, Ltd., and Institute of Psycho-Analysis, 1948.
3. ADLER, ALFRED. Individual Psychology. In: CARL MURCHISON (ed.), Psychologies of 1930, pp. 395–405. Worcester, Mass.: Clark University Press, 1930.
4. A LATE INMATE OF THE GLASGOW ROYAL ASYLUM FOR LUNATICS AT GARTNAVEL. The Philosophy of Insanity. New York: Greenberg Publisher, 1947.
5. ALEXANDER, FRANZ. Fundamentals of Psychoanalysis. New York: W. W. Norton & Co., Inc., 1948.
6. ALEXANDER, FRANZ, et al. Psychoanalytic Therapy: Principles and Application. New York: Ronald Press Co., 1946.
7. ANDREAS-SALOME, LOU. Mein Dank an Freud: Zu Seinem 75. Geburstag. Vienna: Internat. Psychoanal. Verlag, 1931. (Not translated.)
8. BEERS, CLIFFORD. A Mind that Found Itself. New York: Longmans, Green & Co., 1908; Doubleday, Doran & Co., 1945.
9. BENDER, LAURETTA. Techniques of Child Psychiatry. In: BERNARD GLUECK (ed.), Current Therapies of Personality Disorders, pp. 222–41. New York: Grune & Stratton, 1946.
9a. BENEDEK, THERESE. Insight and Personality Adjustment. New York: Ronald Press Co., 1948.
10. BERGLER, EDMUND. The Basic Neurosis. New York: Grune & Stratton, 1949.
11. BLEULER, EUGEN. Textbook of Psychiatry. New York: Macmillan Co., 1924.
12. BINGER, CARL. More about Psychiatry. Chicago: University of Chicago Press, 1949.
13. BINSWANGER, LUDWIG. Grundformen und Erkenntnis menschlichen Daseins. Zurich: Max Niehans Verlag, 1942.

14. BOEHM, FELIX. Paper on the Oedipus Complex, Presented before the German Psychoanalytic Association, Dresden, 1926, Internat. Ztschr. f. Psychoanal., 12:66–79, 1926. (Not translated.)

15. BOISEN, ANTON T. The Exploration of the Inner World. Chicago and New York: Willett, Clark & Co., 1936.

16. BRILL, A. A. Basic Principles of Psychoanalysis. New York: Doubleday & Co., Inc., 1949.

17. BRUCH, HILDE. Puberty and Adolescence: Psychologic Considertions. In: SAM ZACHARY LEVINE et al. (eds.), Advances in Pediatrics, 3:219–90. New York: Interscience Publishers, Inc., 1948.

18. CHICAGO INSTITUTE FOR PSYCHOANALYSIS. The Influence of Psychologic Factors upon Gastro-Intestinal Disturbances: A Symposium, Psychoanalyt. Quart., 3:501–88, 1934.

19. DEUTSCH, FELIX. Analysis of Postural Behavior, Psychoanalyt. Quart., 16:195–213, 1947.

20. DEUTSCH, HELENE. Psychology of Women, Part II: Motherhood. New York: Grune & Stratton, 1946.

21. DIETHELM, OSKAR. Treatment in Psychiatry. New York: Macmillan Co., 1936.

22. DUNBAR, H. FLANDERS. Emotions and Bodily Changes. New York: Columbia University Press, 1938.

23. ———. Synopsis of Psychosomatic Diagnosis and Treatment. New York: Columbia University Press, 1948.

24. EISENBUD, JULE. The Psychology of Headache, Psychiatric Quart., 11:592–619, 1937.

25. ENGLISH, O. SPURGEON. Observation of Trends in Manic-Depressive Psychosis, Psychiatry, 12:125–34, 1949.

26. FAIRBAIRN, W. R. D. Endopsychic Structure Considered in Terms of Object Relationships, Internat. J. Psycho-Analysis, 25:70–93, 1944.

27. ———. Object Relationships and Dynamic Structure, ibid., 27:30–37, 1946.

28. FEDERN, PAUL. Principles of Psychotherapy in Latent Schizophrenia, Am. J. Psychotherapy, 1:129–44, 1947.

29. ———. Psychoanalysis of Psychoses, Psychiatric Quart., 17:3–19, 246–57, 480–87, 1943.

30. FENICHEL, OTTO. Outline of Clinical Psychoanalysis. New York: W. W. Norton & Co., Inc., 1934.

31. ———. Problems of Psychoanalytic Technique, Psychoanalyt. Quart., 7:421–42, 1938; 8:57–87, 164–85, 303–24, 438–70, 1939.

32. FERENCZI, SANDOR. Das Problem der Beendigung der Analysen, Internat. Ztschr. f. Psychoanal., 14:1–10, 1928. Brief translation: On Ending the Analysis, Psychoanalyt. Rev., 15:97–98, 1928.

33. FERENCZI, SANDOR, and RANK, OTTO. The Development of Psychoanalysis. New York and Washington: Nervous and Mental Disease Pub. Co., 1925.

34. FRANK, LAWRENCE K. Family Guidance as an Aspect of Psychiatric Practice. In: BERNARD GLUECK (ed.), Current Therapies of Personality Disorders, pp. 281–91. New York: Grune & Stratton, 1946.

35. FREUD, ANNA. Introduction to the Technic of Child-Analysis. New York and Washington: Nervous and Mental Disease Pub. Co., 1928.

36. ———. The Ego and the Mechanisms of Defence. New York: International Universities Press, Inc., 1946.

37. FREUD, SIGMUND. A General Introduction to Psychoanalysis, chapter on General Theory of the Neuroses. New York: Liveright Pub. Corp., 1935; Garden City Pub. Co., 1943.

38. ———. Chapters on Transference and on The Analytic Therapy, *ibid.*

39. ———. The Dynamics of the Transference. In: Collected Papers, 2:312–22. London: Hogarth Press, 1946.

40. ———. Further Recommendations in the Technique of Psychoanalysis: Observations on Transference-Love. In: Collected Papers, 2:377–91. London: Hogarth Press, 1946.

41. ———. On Psychotherapy. In: Collected Papers, 1:249–63. London: Hogarth Press, 1946.

42. ———. Analysis, Terminable or Interminable, Internat. J. Psycho-Analysis, 18:373–405, 1937.

43. ———. Beyond the Pleasure Principle. London: Hogarth Press, Ltd., and Institute of Psycho-Analysis, 1942.

44. ———. Mourning and Melancholia. In: Collected Papers, 4:152–70. London: Hogarth Press, 1946.

45. ———. Neurosis and Psychosis. In: Collected Papers, 2:250–54. London: Hogarth Press, 1948.

46. ———. New Introductory Lectures on Psychoanalysis, chapter on Explanations, Applications and Orientations, pp. 186–215. New York: W. W. Norton & Co., Inc., 1933.

47. ———. On Narcissism: An Introduction. In: Collected Papers, 4:30–59. London: Hogarth Press, 1946.

48. ———. Psycho-analytic Notes upon an Autobiographical Account of Paranoia (Dementia Paranoides). In: Collected Papers, 3:390–466. London: Hogarth Press, 1946.

49. ———. Psychopathology of Every Day Life. In: The Basic Writings of Sigmund Freud. New York: Modern Library, Random House, Inc., 1938.

50. ———. The Ego and the Id. London: Hogarth Press, Ltd., and Institute of Psycho-Analysis, 1935.

51. ———. The History of the Psychoanalytic Movement. In: The Basic Writings of Sigmund Freud. New York: Modern Library, Random House, Inc., 1938.

52. FREUD, SIGMUND. The Interpretation of Dreams. New York: Macmillan Co., 1931. Also in The Basic Writings of Sigmund Freud. New York: Modern Library, Random House, Inc., 1938.

53. ———. The Passing of the Oedipus-Complex. In: Collected Papers, 2:269–76. London: Hogarth Press, 1948.

54. ———. The Problem of Anxiety. New York: W. W. Norton & Co., 1936.

55. ———. Three Contributions to the Theory of Sex. New York and Washington: Nervous and Mental Disease Pub. Co., 1920.

56. FROMM, ERICH. Escape from Freedom. New York and Toronto: Farrar & Rinehart, Inc., 1947.

57. ———. Man for Himself. New York and Toronto: Rinehart & Co., Inc., 1947.

58. ———. Selfishness and Self-love, Psychiatry, 2:507–23, 1939.

59. ———. The Nature of Dreams, Scient. Am., 180:44–47, 1949.

60. ———. The Oedipus Complex and the Oedipus Myth. In: RUTH NANDA ANSHEN (ed.), The Family: Its Function and Destiny, pp. 334–58. New York: Harper & Bros., 1949.

61. FROMM-REICHMANN, FRIEDA. Contribution to the Psychogenesis of Migraine, Psychoanalyt. Rev., 24:26–33, 1937.

62. ———. Notes on the Mother Role in the Family Group. Bull. Menninger Clin., 4:132–48, 1940.

63. ———. Recent Advances in Psychoanalytic Therapy, Psychiatry, 4:161–64, 1941.

64. ———. Recent Advances in Psychoanalysis, J. Am. M. Women's A., 4:320–26, 1949.

65. ———. Psychoanalytic Psychotherapy with Psychotics, Psychiatry, 6:277–79, 1943.

66. ———. Transference Problems in Schizophrenics, Psychoanalyt. Quart., 8:412–26, 1939.

67. ———. A Preliminary Note on the Emotional Significance of Stereotypies in Schizophrenics, Bull. Forest Sanitarium, 1:17–21, 1942.

68. ———. Notes on the Development of Treatment of Schizophrenics by Psychoanalytic Psychotherapy, Psychiatry, 11:263–73, 1948.

69. ———. Problems of Therapeutic Management in a Psychoanalytic Hospital, Psychoanalyt. Quart., 16:325–56, 1947.

70. ———. Remarks on the Philosophy of Mental Disorder, Psychiatry, 9:293–308, 1946.

71. ———. Intensive Psychotherapy of Manic-depressives, Confinia neurol., 9:158–65, 1949.

72. GLOVER, EDWARD. An Investigation of the Technique of Psychoanalysis. Baltimore: Williams & Wilkins Co., 1940. 2d. ed.: Psycho-analysis: A Handbook. London: Stapler Press, 1948.

73. GOLDSTEIN, KURT. Human Nature in the Light of Psychopathology. Cambridge: Harvard University Press, 1940.

74. ———. The Organism. New York: American Book Co., 1939.

75. GRODDECK, GEORGE. The Book of the It. New York: Funk & Wagnalls Co., 1950; London: C. W. Daniel Co., 1928.
76. ———. Exploring the Unconscious. London: C. W. Daniel Co., 1929.
77. ———. The Unknown Self. London: C. W. Daniel Co., 1929.
78. ———. The World of Man. London: C. W. Daniel Co., 1934.
79a. HARTMANN, H.; KRIS, E.; and LOEWENSTEIN, R. Comments on the Formation of Psychic Structure. In: PHYLLIS GREENACRE et al. (eds.), The Psychoanalytic Study of the Child, Vol. 2. New York: International Universities Press, 1946.
79. HENDRICK, IVES. Facts and Theories of Psychoanalysis. New York: Alfred A. Knopf, 1934.
80. HINSIE, LELAND E. Concepts and Problems of Psychotherapy. New York: Columbia University Press, 1937.
81. ———. The Person in the Body. New York: W. W. Norton & Co., Inc., 1945.
82. ———. Understandable Psychiatry. New York: Macmillan Co., 1938.
83. HORNEY, KAREN. On the Genesis of the Castration Complex in Women. Internat. J. Psycho-Analysis, 5: 50–65, 1924.
84. ———. New Ways in Psychoanalysis, chapter on Psychoanalytic Therapy, pp. 276–305. New York: W. W. Norton & Co., Inc., 1939.
85. ———. The Neurotic Personality of Our Time. New York: W. W. Norton & Co., Inc., 1937.
86. HUTCHINSON, ELIOT D. The Nature of Insight, and Varieties of Insight in Humans. In: PATRICK MULLAHY (ed.), A Study of Interpersonal Relations, pp. 421–45, 386–403. New York: Hermitage Press, Inc., 1949.
87. ISAACS, SUSAN. The Nursery Years. New York: Vanguard Press, 1936.
88. JONES, ERNEST. Papers on Psychoanalysis. Baltimore: Williams & Wilkins Co., 1948.
89. JUNG, CARL G. The Psychology of Dementia Praecox, pp. 10–11, 22, 82–83. ("Nervous and Mental Disease Monographs," No. 3.) New York: Nervous and Mental Disease Pub. Co., 1936.
90. ———. Psychology of the Unconscious: A Study of the Transformations and Symbolisms of the Libido. New York: Moffat, Yard & Co., 1916.
91. KEMPF, E. J. Psychopathology. St. Louis: C. V. Mosby Co., 1920.
92. KLEIN, MELANIE. A Contribution to the Psychogenesis of Manic-depressive States. In: Contributions to Psychoanalysis, 1921–1945, pp. 282–311. London: Hogarth Press and Institute of Psycho-Analysis, 1948.
93. KUBIE, LAWRENCE S. Practical and Theoretical Aspects of Psychoanalysis. New York: International Universities Press, Inc., 1950.

94. LEE, HENRY B. Projective Features of Contemplative Artistic Experience, Am. J. Orthopsychiat., 19: 101–11, 1949.

95. LEVINE, MAURICE. Psychotherapy in Medical Practice. New York: Macmillan Co., 1942.

96. LEVY, JOHN, and MUNROE, RUTH. The Happy Family. New York: Alfred A. Knopf, 1938.

97. LIEBMAN, JOSHUA L. Peace of Mind. New York: Simon & Schuster, 1946.

98. LIEF, ALFRED. The Commonsense Psychiatry of Dr. Adolf Meyer. New York and London: McGraw-Hill Book Co., Inc., 1948.

99. LORAND, SANDOR. Technique of Psychoanalytic Therapy. New York: International Universities Press, 1946.

100. MACK BRUNSWICK, RUTH. A Supplement to Freud's "History of an Infantile Neurosis," Internat. J. Psycho-Analysis, 19:439–76, 1928.

101. MARSH, EARLE M.; MOORE, WILLIAM G.; and VOLLMER, ALBERT M. Your Baby Is Born. San Francisco: Accommodation Letter Shop, 1949.

102. MASSERMAN, JULES H. Principles of Dynamic Psychiatry. Vol. 1. New York: W. B. Saunders Co., 1946.

103. MEAD, MARGARET. Male and Female: A Study of the Sexes in a Changing World. New York: William Morrow & Co., 1949.

104. MENNINGER, KARL A. Love against Hate. New York: Harcourt, Brace & Co., 1942.

105. ———. Man against Himself. New York: Harcourt, Brace & Co., 1938.

106. ———. Psychoanalytic Psychiatry: Theory and Practice, Bull. Menninger Clin., 4: 105–23, 1940.

107. ———. The Human Mind. New York: Alfred A. Knopf, 1946.

108. MENNINGER, WILLIAM C. Psychiatry: Its Evolution and Present Status. Ithaca, N.Y.: Cornell University Press, 1948.

109. MULLAHY, PATRICK. Oedipus Myth and Complex. New York: Hermitage Press, Inc., 1948.

110. MUNCIE, WENDELL. Psychobiology and Psychiatry: A Textbook of Normal and Abnormal Behavior. St. Louis: C. V. Mosby Co., 1948.

111. NUNBERG, HERMAN. Allgemeine Neurosenlehre auf psychoanalytischer Grundlage. Bern: Hans Huber Verlag, 1932. (Not translated.)

112. Panel Discussion on Countertransferences and Attitudes of the Analyst in the Therapeutic Process, Bull. Am. Psychoanalyt. A., 5:46–49, 1949.

113. Panel Discussion on Psychoanalysis of the Creative Imagination, ibid., 4:39–44, 1948.

114. Panel Discussion on the Theory and Treatment of Schizophrenia, ibid., pp. 15–20.

115. PAYNE, SYLVIA. Notes on Developments in the Theory and Prac-

tice of Psychoanalytic Technique, Internat. J. Psycho-Analysis, 27:12–19, 1946.

116. PRESTON, GEORGE H. Psychiatry for the Curious. New York and Toronto: Rinehart & Co., Inc., 1940.

117. ———. The Substance of Mental Health. New York and Toronto: Rinehart & Co., Inc., 1943.

118. Proceedings of the Brief Psychotherapy Council. Chicago: Chicago Institute for Psychoanalysis, 1942.

119. Psychoanalysis Today. Ed. SANDOR LORAND. New York: International Universities Press, 1944.

120. RADO, SANDOR. Developments in the Psychoanalytic Conception and Treatment of the Neuroses, Psychoanalyt. Quart., 8:427–37, 1939.

121. ———. The Problem of Melancholia, Internat. J. Psycho-Analysis, 9:420–38, 1928.

122. ———. The Psychoanalysis of Pharmacothymia (Drug Addiction), Psychoanalyt. Quart., 2:1–23, 1933.

123. RANK, OTTO. Eine Neurosenanalyse in Träumen. Leipzig, Vienna, and Zurich: Internat. Psychoanalyt. Verlag, 1924. (Not translated.)

124. RANK, OTTO, and SACHS, HANNS. Gemeinsame Tagträume. Vienna and Zurich: Internat. Psychoanalyt. Verlag, 1926. (Not translated.)

125. ———. Die Bedeutung der Psychoanalyse für die Geisteswissenschaften, chaps. i and ii. Wiesbaden: J. F. Bergmann, 1913. (Not translated.)

126. RAPAPORT, DAVID. Diagnostic Psychological Testing, Vols. 1 and 2. Chicago: Year Book Publishers, Inc., 1945 and 1946.

127. READ, GRANTLY DICK. Childbirth without Fear. New York and London: Harper & Bros., 1944.

128. REICH, WILHELM. Character-Analysis. New York: Orgone Institute Press, 1949.

129. ———. The Function of the Orgasm. New York: Farrar, Straus, 1948.

130. REIK, THEODOR. Listening with the Third Ear. New York: Farrar, Straus, 1949.

131. ———. The Original of the "Sleeping Beauty" Discovered, Bull. Menninger Clin., 12:166–67, 1948.

132. RIBBLE, MARGARET. The Rights of Infants. New York: Columbia University Press, 1943.

133. RIOCH, JANET M. The Transference Phenomenon in Psychoanalytic Therapy. In: PATRICK MULLAHY (ed.), A Study of Interpersonal Relations, pp. 80–97. New York: Hermitage Press, Inc., 1949.

134. ROGERS, CARL R. Counseling and Psychotherapy. New York: Houghton Mifflin Co., 1942.

135. ROSEN, JOHN N. A Method of Resolving Acute Catatonic Excite-

ment, Psychiat. Quart., 20:183–98, 1946.

136. ———. The Treatment of Schizophrenic Psychosis by Direct Analytic Therapy, *ibid.*, 21:3–37, 117–19, 1947.

137. SCHACHTEL, ERNEST. On Memory and Childhood Amnesia. In: PATRICK MULLAHY (ed.), A Study of Interpersonal Relations, pp. 3–49. New York: Hermitage Press, Inc., 1949.

138. SCHILDER, PAUL. Psychotherapy. New York: W. W. Norton & Co., Inc., 1938.

139. SHARPE, ELLA. Dream Analysis. London: Hogarth Press, 1938.

140. SILBERER, HERBERT. Der Traum–Einführung in die Traumpsychologie. Stuttgart, 1919. (Not translated.)

141. SILVERBERG, WILLIAM V. The Concept of Transference, Psychoanalyt. Quart., 17:303–21, 1948.

142. SIMMEL, ERNST. Die psychoanalytische Behandlung in der Klinik, Internat. Ztschr. f. Psychoanal., 14:352–70, 1928. Translation: Internat. J. Psycho-Analysis, 10:70–89, 1929.

143. STAVEREN, HERBERT. Suggested Specificity of Certain Dynamisms in a Case of Schizophrenia. In: PATRICK MULLAHY (ed.), A Study of Interpersonal Relations, pp. 455–70. New York: Hermitage Press, Inc., 1949.

144. STEKEL, WILHELM. Interpretation of Dreams. New York: Liveright Pub. Corp., 1943.

145. STERBA, RICHARD. Dreams and Acting Out, Psychoanalyt. Quart., 15:175–79, 1946.

146. Studien über Autorität und Familie. Paris: Librairie Félix Alcan, 1936; New York: Institute of Social Research, 1937. (German with English and French abstracts of each contribution.)

147. SULLIVAN, H. S. Conceptions of Modern Psychiatry. Reprinted from Psychiatry, 3:1–117, 1940; 8:177–205, 1945. Washington, D.C.: William Alanson White Psychiatric Foundation, 1947.

148. ———. Affective Experience in Early Schizophrenia, Am. J. Psychiatry, 6:468–83, 1927.

149. ———. Notes on Investigation, Therapy, and Education in Psychiatry and Their Relations to Schizophrenia, *ibid.*, 10:271–80, 1947.

150. ———. The Meaning of Anxiety in Psychiatry and in Life, *ibid.*, 11:1–13, 1948.

151. ———. The Theory of Anxiety and the Nature of Psychotherapy, *ibid.*, 12:3–12, 1949.

152. ———. The Study of Psychiatry: Three Orienting Lectures, *ibid.*, 10:355–71, 1947.

153. TAUSK, VICTOR. Zwei homosexuelle Träume, Internat. Ztschr. f. Psychoanal., 2:36–39, 1914. (Not translated.)

154. The Proceedings of the Third Psychotherapy Council. Chicago: R. R. Donnelley & Sons Co., 1947.

155. THOMPSON, CLARA. Development of Awareness of Transference in a Markedly Detached Personality, Internat. J. Psycho-Analysis, 19:299, 1938.

156. ———. Transference as a Therapeutic Instrument. In: BERNARD GLUECK (ed.), Current Therapies of Personality Disorders, pp. 194–205. New York: Grune & Stratton, 1946.

157. ———. Ferenczi's Contribution to Psychoanalysis, Psychiatry, 7:245–52, 1944.

158. ———. The Therapeutic Technique of Sandor Ferenczi: A Comment, Internat. J. Psycho-Analysis, 24:64–66, 1943.

159. ———. "Penis Envy" in Women, Psychiatry, 6:123–25, 1943.

160. TOWER, SARAH S. Management of Paranoid Trends in Treatment of a Post-psychotic Obsessional Condition. In: PATRICK MULLAHY (ed.), A Study of Interpersonal Relations, pp. 471–79. New York: Hermitage Press, Inc., 1949.

161. WEIGERT, EDITH V. Dissent in the Early History of Psychoanalysis, Psychiatry, 5:349–59, 1942.

162. ———. Existentialism and Its Relation to Psychotherapy, ibid., 12:399–412, 1949.

163. WEISS and ENGLISH. Psychosomatic Medicine. Philadelphia and London: W. B. Saunders Co., 1943.

164. WHITE, WILLIAM ALANSON. Medical Philosophy, Psychiatry, 10:77–98, 191–210, 1947.

165. ———. Medical Psychology: The Mental Factor in Disease. New York and Washington: Nervous and Mental Disease Pub. Co., 1931.

166. ———. Outlines of Psychiatry. Washington: Nervous and Mental Disease Pub. Co., 1935.

167. ———. The Autobiography of a Purpose. New York: Doubleday, Doran & Co., 1938.

168. WHITEHORN, JOHN C. Psychotherapy. In: NOEL G. HARRIS (ed.), Modern Trends in Psychological Medicine, chap. x. New York: Paul B. Hoeber, Inc., 1948; London: Butterworth & Co., 1948.

169. ———. Sex Behavior and Sex Attitudes in Relation to Emotional Health, Stanford M. Bull., 7:45–60, 93–99, 1949.

170. WILHELM, RICHARD. Das Geheimnis der goldenen Blüte with a commentary by C. G. Jung. Munich: Dornverlag Grete Ullmann, 1929. (Not translated.)

171. WOLFF, HAROLD. Headache and Other Head Pain. London and New York: Oxford University Press, 1948.

172. ZILBOORG, GREGORY. Considerations on Suicide with Particular Reference to That of the Young, Am. J. Orthopsychiat., 7:15–31, 1937.

173. ———. Differential Diagnostic Types of Suicide, Arch. Neurol. and Psychiat., 35:270–91, 1936.

174. ———. Psychiatric Perspectives of Today, Bull. N.Y. Acad. Med., 25:577–86, 1949.

175. ———. Suicide among Civilized and Primitive Races, Am. J. Psychiat., 92:1347–69, 1936.

# INDEX

# INDEX

For authors not mentioned in the Index consult Reference List, pp. 227–35.

[ 239 ]